Ricardo Navas

Ricardo Navas

Comprehensive Manuals of Surgical Specialties

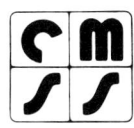

Richard H. Egdahl, editor

Bradley J. Harlan   Albert Starr   Fredric M. Harwin

Manual of Cardiac Surgery
Volume II

Includes 130 illustrations in full color

Springer-Verlag
New York   Heidelberg   Berlin

SERIES EDITOR

Richard H. Egdahl, M.D., Ph.D., Professor of Surgery, Boston University Medical Center, Boston, Massachusetts 02118

AUTHORS

Bradley J. Harlan, M.D., Associate Professor of Surgery, Division of Cardiopulmonary Surgery, University of Oregon Health Sciences Center, Portland, Oregon 97201

Albert Starr, M.D., Professor of Surgery and Chief of Division of Cardiopulmonary Surgery, University of Oregon Health Sciences Center, Portland, Oregon 97201

Fredric M. Harwin, B.F.A., M.S., Medical Illustrator, 9101 S. W. 15th Avenue, Portland, Oregon 97219

CONTRIBUTORS

Alain Carpentier, M.D., Professor of Cardiac Surgery, Hôpital Broussais, University of Paris, Paris, France

Professor Lucio Parenzan, M.D., Chief, Cardiac Surgery, Ospedali Riuniti, Bergamo, Italy

Magdi H. Yacoub, F.R.C.S., Consultant Cardiac Surgeon, Harefield Hospital and National Heart Hospital, London, England

MEDICAL PHOTOGRAPHER

Paul Ramsey, 2443 N.E. 20th Street, Portland, Oregon 97212

Sponsoring Editor: Larry W. Carter
Production: Berta Steiner
Design: Caliber Design Planning, Inc.

Library of Congress Cataloging in Publication Data
Harlan, Bradley J.
    Manual of cardiac surgery.

    (Comprehensive manuals of surgical specialities)
    Includes bibliographies and index.
    1. Heart—Surgery. I. Starr, Albert, 1926-   joint author. II. Harwin, Fredric M., joint author.
III. Cardiac surgery. IV. Title. [DNLM: 1. Heart surgery. WG169 H283m 1980]
RD598.H32   617'.412   80-18213
ISBN 0-387-90393-3 (v. 1)   AACR1
ISBN 0-387-90563-4 (v. 2)

© 1981 by Springer-Verlag New York Inc.
All rights reserved. No part of this book may be translated or reproduced in any form without written permission from Springer-Verlag, 175 Fifth Avenue, New York, New York 10010, U.S.A.

The use of general descriptive names, trade names, trademarks, etc. in this publication, even if the former are not especially identified, is not to be taken as a sign that such names, as understood by the Trade Marks and Merchandise Marks Act, may accordingly be used freely by anyone.

Printed in the United States of America.

9 8 7 6 5 4 3 2 1

ISBN 0-387-90563-4   Springer-Verlag New York Heidelberg Berlin
ISBN 3-540-90563-4   Springer-Verlag Berlin Heidelberg New York

To our families and loved ones,
whose gracious acceptance
of the demands of our surgical and artistic lives
made these volumes possible

Contents

Editor's Note
(Richard H. Egdahl) xi

Prefaces xiii

14 Aortic Valve Surgery 205

Valvotomy 205
Replacement 206
Surgical Relief of Other Forms of Left Ventricular Outflow
 Obstruction 226

15 Left Ventricular Aneurysm 233

Resection 233

16 Postinfarction Ventricular Septal Defect 242

Indications 242
Surgical Strategy 242
Surgical Anatomy 243
Technique 243
Results 245

17 Tricuspid Valve Surgery 247

Anuloplasty 247
Commissurotomy 252
Replacement 253

18 Pulmonary Valve Stenosis 256

Pulmonary Valvotomy 256

19 Atrial Septal Defects 261

Indications for Surgery 261
Sinus Venosus Defect 262
Ostium Secundum Defects 264
Ostium Primum Defect 266

20 Complete Atrioventricular Canal 269

Indications for Surgery 269
Surgical Strategy 269
Surgical Anatomy 270
Surgical Technique 270
Results 274

21 Ventricular Septal Defects 276

Indications for Surgery 276
Choice of Operation 277
Surgical Strategy 277
Surgical Anatomy 278
Surgical Technique 280

22 Tetralogy of Fallot 288

Indications 288
Surgical Strategy 290
Surgical Anatomy 292
Technique 293
Late Results 298

23 Transposition of the Great Arteries 302

(Coauthored by Lucio Parenzan and Magdi Yacoub)

Indications for Surgery 303
Choice of Corrective Operation 205
Surgical Strategy 306
Mustard Operation 307
Senning Operation 317
Anatomic Correction 321

24 Total Anomalous Pulmonary Venous Connection 333

Indications for Surgery 333
Surgical Strategy 333
Supracardiac Type 333
Cardiac Type 337
Infracardiac Type 339
Results 340

Index 343

Editor's Note

Comprehensive Manuals of Surgical Specialties is a series of surgical manuals designed to present current operative techniques and to explore various aspects of diagnosis and treatment. The series features a unique format with emphasis on large, detailed, full-color illustrations, schematic charts, and photographs to demonstrate integral steps in surgical procedures.

Each manual focuses on a specific region or topic and describes surgical anatomy, physiology, pathology, diagnosis, and operative treatment. Operative techniques and stratagems for dealing with surgically correctable disorders are described in detail. Illustrations are primarily depicted from the surgeon's viewpoint to enhance clarity and comprehension.

Other volumes in the series:

Published:

Manual of Endocrine Surgery
Manual of Burns
Manual of Surgery of the Gallbladder, Bile Ducts, and Exocrine Pancreas
Manual of Gynecologic Surgery
Manual of Urologic Surgery
Manual of Lower Gastrointestinal Surgery
Manual of Vascular Surgery, Volume I
Manual of Cardiac Surgery, Volume I
Manual of Liver Surgery

In Preparation:

Manual of Vascular Surgery, Volume II
Manual of Soft Tissue Tumor Surgery
Manual of Orthopedic Surgery
Manual of Chest Surgery
Manual of Upper Gastrointestinal Surgery
Manual of Ambulatory Surgery
Manual of Trauma Surgery

Richard H. Egdahl

Prefaces

This second volume of the *Manual of Cardiac Surgery* describes aortic valve surgery, tricuspid valve surgery, surgery for ventricular aneurysm and postinfarction ventricular septal defect, and operations for congenital diseases requiring cardiopulmonary bypass. Volume I covered remaining operations for acquired and congenital cardiac disease and perioperative care.

We have tried to be as detailed as possible regarding the process of cardiac surgery, from coverage of basic surgical technique—an important but frequently ignored subject—to careful description of every essential step of each operation. Carefully conceived and superbly executed full-color illustrations are the primary vehicle for conveying this information. We have not shown all possible methods of performing each operation. The choice of techniques is somewhat arbitrary, but those chosen are the ones developed over two decades of clinical practice and resident training at the University of Oregon Health Sciences Center. These techniques have served us well.

The text authors are proud to have the illustrator, Mr. Fredric Harwin, as coauthor. Mr. Harwin has been a significant contributor to the basic concepts and intellectual substance of the book. His art is a powerful instrument of education.

It is hoped that this book will have broad appeal to all persons caring for cardiac surgical patients. If it increases knowledge and understanding of cardiac surgery and thereby improves patient care, it will have met its main objective.

Bradley J. Harlan, M.D.
Albert Starr, M.D.

A medical illustrator must understand the philosophies and techniques of the scientist as well as those of the artist. This blending has rendered my special interest, the expression of surgical technique, exciting and rewarding to me as a visual communicator.

To illustrate both volumes of *Manual of Cardiac Surgery*, it was necessary to develop an illustrative technique that would allow the audience to visualize accurately the surgical field, where observation is limited and orientation difficult, to represent it as the surgeon sees it, and to understand the anatomy, which is not always visible. In part, this was accomplished by painting on both surfaces of transparent paper to create the illusion of looking through superficial layers to the deeper structures. A combination of color media, including colored pencil, graphite, carbon, pastels, and transparent and opaque watercolors, enabled me to convey the field with minimal loss of reality or dimension.

Of equal importance was the availability, for every illustration, of direct surgical observation, surgical photographs, fresh specimens, and the surgical instruments. The sequence of creation was first the discussion of desired illustrations, then a rough sketch, consultation with the surgeons, finished pencil drawing, another consultation, and finally the color rendering. These color renderings were then checked against actual surgery for accuracy in representation of tissues, instrumentation, tissue responses to manipulation, and consistency of representation. From these processes evolved a technique that facilitated the flow of information, in logical sequence, from one step to the next and from one procedure to another, always focusing the attention of the audience toward what is pertinent and away from the extraneous.

Very close communication between artist and surgeon is necessary to produce illustrations that are both anatomically and surgically correct and artistically viable. Such communication was present during the preparation of this volume, as the text authors and the illustration author cooperated to convey not only the fundamentals of the operations, but also their most subtle details.

Fredric M. Harwin

Acknowledgments

We wish to thank our colleagues at the University of Oregon Health Sciences Center and elsewhere who directly and indirectly inspired many of the concepts of this book and provided valuable review of the manuscript. The concepts and practices described are the result of the interplay of many residents over the years, as well as the constant interchange of ideas with the other staff members of the Division of Cardiopulmonary Surgery, Siavosh Khonsari, James A. Wood, Richard D. Chapman, Aftab Ahmad, and G. Hugh Lawrence. In addition, we thank Martin Lees, Cecille Sunderland, and Henry Issenberg, from the Division of Pediatric Cardiology, who reviewed portions of the manuscript.

The creation of the illustrations was enhanced by the excellent photographs of our operations taken by Mr. Paul Ramsey. McAlpine's superb book, *Heart and Coronary Arteries,* helped greatly in creation of the anatomic illustrations. Dr. Nelson R. Niles, from our Department of Pathology, has also helped by providing specimens for anatomic study.

We wish to thank Dr. Richard H. Egdahl for asking us to participate in this series. We are grateful for the secretarial work of Edie Stout, Ursula Jahns, and Sharon Harlan. Once again, our thanks to Springer-Verlag and their superb staff. We consider ourselves fortunate to be beneficiaries of Springer-Verlag's longstanding expertise in the field of color reproduction and their strong commitment to quality.

Aortic Valve Surgery

14

Surgery of the aortic valve spans all age groups and encompasses a broad spectrum of pathologic anatomy and surgical technique. In this chapter we will illustrate aortic valvotomy and replacement and briefly review surgical relief of other forms of left ventricular outflow obstruction.

Valvotomy

Indications

The indications for aortic valvotomy differ according to age group. Congestive heart failure is the main indication for surgery in infancy, whereas prevention of sudden death and relief of symptoms are the main indications in childhood.[5,41,64] Valvotomy should be performed in any infant in congestive failure and should be performed in any child with critical aortic stenosis, regardless of symptoms. Although the criteria should not be rigid, severe aortic stenosis is indicated by a systolic pressure gradient exceeding 75 mm Hg in the presence of normal cardiac output or a valve area index less than 0.5 cm^2/m^2.

Surgical Anatomy

Congenital aortic stenosis occurs most commonly as a relative underdevelopment of the right coronary cusp and fusion with the adjacent cusps at the commissures. The orifice is usually a slit between the left and noncoronary cusps, and the commissure between these two cusps is usually wide open. One fused commissure of the right coronary cusp is usually well developed, whereas the other commissure can vary in degree of development and may be only a primitive raphe. A safe incision can usually be made in at least one commissure of the right coronary cusp. Incision of the other commissure depends upon its degree of development and the development and depth of the right coronary cusp.

Technique

A transverse aortotomy is made and the valve is exposed with small leaflet retractors. With forceps holding the leaflets, the well-developed commissure is incised back to the anulus (Figs. 14-1, 14-2). The depth of support and degree of development of the right coronary cusp are then assessed. If it is clear that the right coronary cusp will coapt with the other cusps rather than prolapse, the other commissure is incised. Following valvotomy the subvalvular area should be inspected to ensure the absence of any subvalvular stenosis.

Results

Although valvotomy is associated with high operative mortality in the neonate, survivors have good relief of congestive heart failure and good late survival.[33] A large proportion of patients who die may constitute an intermediate group between patients with "hypoplastic left-heart syndrome" and normals,[33] but further studies are needed in this area.

Valvotomy in children has low operative risk, produces excellent symptomatic improvement, but does not usually eliminate the valvular gradient entirely.[24,55,65] Conkle and co-workers[24] reported 38 patients operated upon between 1 and 21 years of age. Ninety percent were asymptomatic. The average mean gradient was reduced from 91 mm Hg to 27 mm Hg. Lawson and colleagues,[65] from the University of Oregon, reported 44 patients, with a mean age at surgery of 10 years. Ninety-two percent survived 10 years and 82% were reoperation-free at 10 years. After 10 years reoperation becomes increasingly common, being performed for either restenosis or progressive regurgitation.

Replacement

Indications

Aortic Stenosis

The natural history of severe aortic stenosis in the adult is markedly unfavorable, with a mortality of 8%–9% per year.[39,92] With the onset of angina the life expectancy is five years, with syncope it is three years. The onset of congestive heart failure carries the worst prognosis, with an average life expectancy of less than two years.[100] Proper timing of aortic valve replacement prevents early and late death, results in normal functional status, and preserves normal ventricular function or returns abnormal function to normal. Knowledge of how the natural course is altered by properly timed and properly performed valve replacement forms the basis for decision regarding surgical intervention.

Aortic stenosis is usually a progressive disease. The increasing resistance to left ventricular outflow caused by progressive stenosis of the aortic valve is compensated by the generation of increasingly higher left ventricular pressure in order to maintain adequate systemic pressure and cardiac output. This increased left ventricular pressure is achieved by concentric ventricular hypertrophy, with thickening of the left ventricular wall and increase in mass of the left ventricle.[36,49,84] Such hypertrophy normalizes wall stress and initially maintains normal left ventricular systolic pump function.[34,47,48]

However, the ventricle may reach a limit of concentric hypertrophy and begin to dilate, using the Frank-Starling mechanism in order to maintain left ventricular systolic pump function. The dilatation and change in shape are critical developments in the decompensation of ventricular function. Parameters of systolic pump function such as ejection fraction and mean velocity

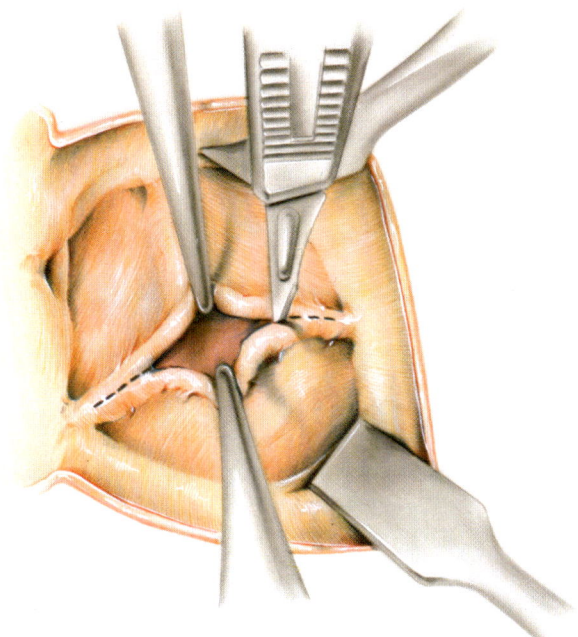
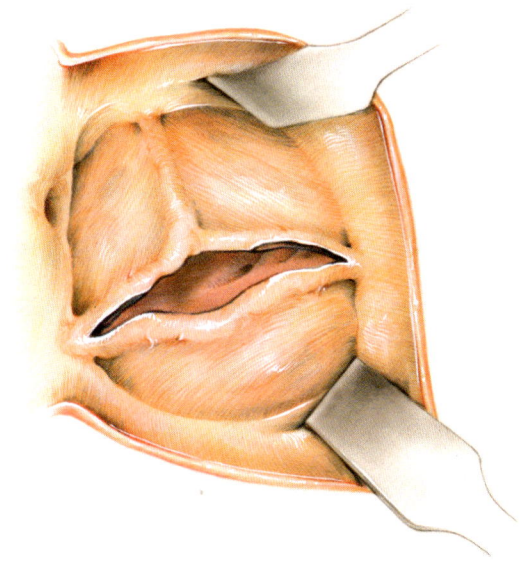

FIGURE 14-1   FIGURE 14-2

of circumferential fiber shortening may be maintained initially in the normal range,[99] but subsequently are reduced in all, and eventually congestive heart failure results.

Hemodynamic and metabolic alterations are the consequence of these progressive stages of left ventricular compensation and then decompensation; the hemodynamic and metabolic changes cause the symptoms and events characteristic of aortic stenosis. As the ventricular compliance falls with increasing hypertrophy, the end-diastolic pressure and pulmonary venous pressure rise. This can cause increasing shortness of breath. As the myocardial wall tension increases and the oxygen demand rises, an imbalance between oxygen supply and demand may occur, resulting in myocardial ischemia and the symptom of angina pectoris. The presence of coronary artery disease will cause myocardial ischemia earlier in the course of the disease.

Transient periods of systemic hypotension may occur, resulting in dizziness or syncope. Sudden death may occur, probably most commonly caused by ventricular arrhythmias secondary to myocardial ischemia. Chronic congestive heart failure develops as decompensation progresses, with the alteration in ventricular shape and dynamics creating a vicious cycle, terminating in death if surgical treatment does not ensue.

Surgical intervention in aortic stenosis should be timed to relieve symptoms, prevent or reverse ventricular dysfunction, and prevent cardiac death. This timing can be determined with assurance since the results for surgical treatment of severe aortic stenosis are clearly superior to the natural history.[4,84,109,112] Valve replacement for aortic stenosis results in alleviation of symptoms and improvement in ventricular function in the vast majority of patients. Even those patients with congestive heart failure and marked deterioration of ventricular function usually have marked improvement in symptoms and ventricular function,[109] illustrating the reversibility of the ventricular dysfunction occurring from aortic stenosis. However, in this group late death following successful valve replacement is more common.

Because of the poor prognosis of severe aortic stenosis and the good results of surgical treatment, surgery should be performed if severe stenosis is documented by catheterization, regardless of the frequency or severity of symptoms. Hemodynamic evaluation in our institution involves determination of the valvular gradient and calculation of the aortic valve area and the aortic valve area index. In the presence of a normal ejection fraction and cardiac output, a gradient of 50 mm Hg or more usually correlates with severe aortic stenosis (aortic valve area index less than 0.75 cm^2/m^2). If cardiac output is low, severe aortic stenosis may exist without a high gradient.[20] It is for this reason that valve area index is calculated.

Aortic Regurgitation

Acute aortic regurgitation, as can occur with endocarditis or dissection of the ascending aorta, can present as sudden hemodynamic deterioration,[92,116,119] requiring urgent surgery. The hemodynamic indications in the face of sudden hemodynamic deterioration are clear and uncontroversial.

However, there is considerable controversy regarding the indications for surgical intervention in chronic aortic regurgitation.[51,82,88,91,105] This reflects both recognition of the inadequacy of the older indications—development of severe symptoms, congestive heart failure, or marked cardiomegaly—and realization that a predictable and widely acceptable new set of indications has not yet been developed.

Aortic valve replacement for chronic aortic regurgitation has generally been less satisfactory than replacement for aortic stenosis, in terms of improvement in symptoms, improvement in ventricular function, and late survival.[4,13,17,22,36,37,44,60] It appears that there are several reasons for this disparity in results: (1) aortic regurgitation usually does not cause symptoms until considerable ventricular dysfunction has developed;[36,43] (2) the ventricular dysfunction present at the time symptoms develop seldom improves completely to normal following successful valve replacement;[13,44] (3) severe ventricular dysfunction often progresses in spite of successful valve replacement, resulting in late death.[11,50,53]

The major compensatory changes caused by aortic regurgitation are left ventricular hypertrophy and ventricular dilatation.[84] Such compensation can maintain normal ejection fraction and normal end-diastolic pressure for a long period of time, by increasing stroke volume in response to volume overload. Eventually the ejection fraction begins to fall, first only during exercise,[12] then at rest. The left ventricular end-diastolic pressure rises and pulmonary venous hypertension ensues, causing dyspnea and orthopnea. Therefore, with aortic regurgitation, in contrast to aortic stenosis, symptoms usually do not occur until considerable ventricular dysfunction has occurred.[36] Also, the ventricular structural and functional changes occurring with volume overload are more severe and much less reversible than the changes occurring with pressure overload.[71,84,101]

Maron and colleagues[71] have described cardiac muscle degeneration in the left ventricle of patients with pure aortic regurgitation or combined aortic stenosis and regurgitation. These morphologic features are decreased size of cells; loss of myofibrils; preferential loss of thick (myosin) filaments; streaking, streaming and clumping of Z band material; markedly increased amounts of interstitial fibrous tissue; loss of contact between adjacent cells; dilatation or proliferation of sarcoplasmic reticulum; and thickening of the basement membrane. Although their series is small, including only 16 patients, they did not observe any such degeneration in the 6 patients with predominant aortic stenosis.

Experimental work by Ross and colleagues[101] has shown that chronic left ventricular volume overload results in slippage between myofibrils, reflected by a loss of normal alignment of the Z lines. It has been suggested that such a fundamental qualitative change in the microarchitecture of the ventricle with chronic volume overloading may be partially or totally irreversible.[36]

Dissatisfaction with the traditional indications for valve replacement in aortic regurgitation has stimulated search for better parameters upon which to base the timing of surgery. These have involved invasive and noninvasive evaluation of ventricular function, at rest and during stress.

Afterload stress with angiotensin has resulted in a fall in ejection fraction in approximately 50% of patients with aortic regurgitation.[8] The stress-induced dysfunction correlated with a regurgitant fraction over 0.50 and a left ventricular end-diastolic volume index over 160 ml/m^2. Radionuclide cineangiography has demonstrated an abnormal ejection fraction during exercise in almost all patients with aortic regurgitation and in approximately 50% of asymptomatic patients.[12] Measurement of left ventricular function during stress may prove valuable in determining the optimal time for aortic valve replacement.

Echocardiographic studies of left ventricular dimensions have been correlated with postoperative results.[50] Patients with left ventricular end-systolic dimensions below 55 mm usually have good results. It has been recommended that asymptomatic patients with end-systolic dimensions of 50–54 mm be followed with serial echocardiograms every 4–6 months and operation performed at an end-systolic dimension of 55 mm or greater, in spite of absence of symptoms.[51]

Rahimtoola[91] recommends consideration of aortic valve replacement in asymptomatic patients with severe aortic regurgitation and impaired resting left ventricular pump function, stressing that more information is needed before even a tentative conclusion can be reached in patients with normal resting but impaired exercise left ventricular ejection fraction.

We recommend valve replacement in severe aortic regurgitation and impaired resting left ventricular ejection fraction, regardless of symptomatic state. All symptomatic patients with severe aortic regurgitation should undergo valve replacement. The indications for surgical intervention in severe chronic aortic regurgitation will continue to evolve, influenced by improving surgical results, increased knowledge, and the use of new technology for preoperative evaluation.[97,110] The goal should always be to perform surgery before left ventricular dysfunction becomes irreversible.

Combined Stenosis and Regurgitation
Patients with aortic stenosis and regurgitation cover a broad spectrum of physiologic conditions and must be evaluated carefully, since they can have a more rapidly progressive and malignant course, probably due to the early loss of ventricular shape in the presence of outflow obstruction. Patients with symptoms and normal ventricular function should undergo surgery, as should asymptomatic patients with resting left ventricular dysfunction.

Endocarditis
The treatment of endocarditis is primarily medical. The indications for operation in endocarditis are many and varied, depending on the organism, its response to antibiotic treatment, hemodynamic abnormalities, and other factors.[14,75,77,81,89,95,108,113,117] Surgery should be undertaken if there is persistent infection, development of congestive heart failure, septic embolus, or heart block.

Surgery should also be influenced by the type of organism. Fungal endocarditis and most gram-negative infections should indicate early surgery regardless of the hemodynamic state.[14,95,117] Infection with *Staphylococcus aureus* is prone to cause heart failure, anular and myocardial abscesses, heart block, and coronary embolism. Early surgery for staphylococcal endocarditis, regardless of hemodynamic state, has also been recommended.[95] Surgical excision of the focus of infection prior to extension or abscess formation is an advantage of early surgical intervention in medically recalcitrant situations.

Combined with Coronary Artery Surgery
Valvular replacement in the presence of untreated coronary disease is associated with higher early and late mortality than valvular replacement in the absence of coronary disease,[29,67,86] as discussed in Chapter 9. Copeland and co-workers[29] found a three-year survival of 60% in 129 patients with isolated aortic valve replacement who had untreated coronary disease. The three-year survival following isolated aortic valve replacement in 213 patients without coronary artery disease was 85%, a statistically significant difference.

There is good evidence that performing coronary bypass for coronary artery disease at the time of valve replacement improves survival in patients with combined disease if the operative mortality is low (below 6%).[96] It is our policy to perform coronary arteriography in all patients over 40 years of age who have valvular disease.[3,9] Coronary artery bypass is performed to major vessels with over 50% narrowing of luminal diameter. Bypass is done even if angina is not present.

Choice of Prosthesis

The reasoning underlying our choice of type of valvular prosthesis for aortic valve replacement is covered in detail in *Cardiac Valve Prostheses*, by Lefrak and Starr.[66] The current choice, for the most part, is between two widely used types of mechanical prosthesis (ball valve and tilting disc) and the porcine xenograft bioprosthesis.

Mechanical and xenograft prostheses are similar in hemodynamic function in the commonly used sizes, removing hemodynamics as a basis of choice in most instances. However, the porcine xenografts are more likely to produce a "prosthesis-patient mismatch"[90] in the smaller sizes. We try to avoid using an aortic porcine xenograft smaller than 25 mm in the normal-sized adult male.

The main factors affecting choice of prosthesis are anticoagulation and attitude of the patient and surgeon regarding reoperation. Porcine valves have the advantage of a low embolic rate in the absence of anticoagulant therapy if sinus rhythm is present; they have the disadvantage of unproven long-term durability beyond five years, with evidence of increasing leaflet failure after five years.[63] Porcine valves are likely, at some time, to require reoperation due to degeneration and structural failure. The amount of time postimplant that will pass before such degeneration occurs is not known at this time. Therefore we feel the strong possibility of eventual reoperation should be understood and accepted by the patient before a porcine xenograft is implanted.

All mechanical prostheses require continuous anticoagulation. Therefore, patient factors weighing against anticoagulation (previous bleeding history, inability or unwillingness to conform to daily medication and periodic blood tests) favor use of a xenograft valve. If there are no contraindications to anticoagulation and the patient is likely to survive ten or more years following valve replacement, we generally recommend a mechanical ball-valve prosthesis (Silastic ball Starr-Edwards 1260). If the patient prefers not to take anticoagulants and has few qualms about the possibility of reoperation, a bioprosthesis is used.

Newer valvular prostheses will continue to be developed, and our knowledge about present prostheses will grow. The data upon which decisions regarding choice of prosthesis are made will expand. Because of insufficient knowledge, firm conclusions cannot be made at this time. The variables influencing valve selection now and in the immediate future between mechanical and tissue valves are as follows:

1. What is the risk of anticoagulant therapy in a particular patient?
2. Is the patient a reasonable risk for reoperation? How does the patient view that possibility?
3. Is there a pregnancy planned?
4. What is the anticipated life expectancy of the patient? Is it shorter than the known durability of the bioprosthesis?
5. Having made a tentative selection, are there anatomic conditions (size of anulus) at surgery favoring one prosthesis over the other?

Surgical Strategy

Myocardial Preservation
Cold potassium crystalloid cardioplegic arrest is used for aortic valve replacement in most cases (Chapter 6). In patients with end-stage aortic stenosis undergoing isolated valve replacement, there may be some advantage to rapid valve excision and placement of sutures in the anulus, followed by coronary perfusion during the rest of the procedure, providing the total ischemic period is no longer than 10–15 minutes.

Venting
The left ventricle is usually vented through the apex. The vent is on gravity drainage when the aorta is closed and on suction when the aorta is open.

Associated Cardiac Procedures
1. Coronary artery bypass: Distal anastomoses are done after opening the aorta and injecting cardioplegic solution into the coronary ostia via hand-held cannulas. Incisions in the epicardium over the sites of coronary arteriotomy *prior* to infusion of cardioplegic solution can help in assuring accurate incision in the blanched coronary arteries. Following all the distal anastomoses, the aortic anular sutures are placed, the valve inserted, and the aortotomy closed. Proximal vein anastomoses are done over a partial occluding clamp after release of the aortic cross-clamp, while the vented heart is beating and rewarming.

2. Mitral valve replacement: The mitral valve and aortic valve are excised. Sutures are placed in the mitral anulus and through the prosthetic valve. The valve can be seated and tied at this time or after placement of the aortic anular sutures; the latter may give better exposure of the aortic anulus. Sutures are placed through the aortic anulus and prosthetic valve. The mitral valve is then seated and tied, followed by the aortic valve.

Suture Technique
Suture techniques applicable to the aortic valve include (1) simple interrupted, (2) interrupted vertical mattress, (3) interrupted mattress with pledgets,[42,62] and (4) continuous.[27] Our standard technique for use with the Starr-Edwards aortic prosthesis is interrupted vertical mattress. The porcine bioprosthesis is inserted with simple interrupted sutures.

Management of the Small Aortic Anulus
There are two main methods of managing a small aortic anulus: (1) If a moderate increase in anular diameter is required (2–6 mm), the aortic anulus can be divided at the base of the anterior leaflet of the mitral valve and

patch reconstruction performed in conjunction with aortic valve replacement. (2) If a marked increase in anular diameter is desired, the aortic anulus can be divided through the right coronary cusp and into the muscular ventricular septum and right ventricular outflow tract, with patch repair of the ventricular and right ventricular outflow defects performed in conjunction with aortic valve replacement.

Anular enlargement through the anulus at the base of the mitral leaflet involves several variables: (1) location of the anular incision, (2) depth of the anular incision (whether there is extension onto the mitral leaflet and, if so, its depth), (3) whether incision is made into the left atrium, (4) level of valve ring placement, and others.[7,56,70,87,98] Our preferred methods are illustrated in the technique section which follows.

A more radical method of anular enlargement may be required, especially in the child undergoing surgery for congenital aortic stenosis with hypoplastic anulus. A method that permits as much as doubling of the anular diameter has been described by Konno.[61] This procedure involves incising the aortic anulus through the right coronary cusp to the left of the right coronary orifice. The incision is carried into the ventricular septum and into the right ventricular outflow tract. A two-layered Dacron patch is then used to close the ventricular defect. The valve is then inserted and fixed to the patch. One layer of patch is sutured to the right ventricular outflow tract and the other layer is sutured to the aortotomy. This technique of aortoventriculoplasty gives promise of being an effective and safe operation for a difficult anatomic problem.[93]

Management of Anular Erosion or Abscess

Destruction of tissue of the aortic root can present one of the most formidable challenges encountered by the cardiac surgeon. Such destruction usually occurs secondary to *Staph. aureus* endocarditis. The effect is similar to that of a mycotic aneurysm.[45] Erosion or abscess formation can occur into the ventricular septum under the right coronary cusp, between the left or noncoronary cusp and the mitral leaflet, as well as at the junction of the left atrial wall. Erosions can perforate into the right ventricle, right atrium, or pericardium.[18,21]

A number of methods have been described to deal with this serious problem. Closure of the erosions with Teflon strips for buttressing, with pulling together of the erosion as the valve is seated, has been recommended.[19,107,117] Danielson and colleagues[31] have described implantation of an aortic valve prosthesis into the ascending aorta, anastomosis of saphenous vein grafts to the right and left coronary systems, with proximal anastomoses placed above the aortic valve, and closure of the coronary ostia. Frantz and co-workers[40] reported two patients with left ventricular–aortic discontinuity complicating bacterial endocarditis who underwent composite prosthetic valve–Dacron tube graft reconstruction of the aortic root. The prosthetic valve was sutured into the remaining aortic anulus, ventricular muscle, and base of the aortic leaflet of the mitral valve. The coronary arteries were sutured to openings in the side of the graft.

We have not yet encountered a case of anular erosion that appeared to require as extensive an operation as those described by Danielson or Frantz. Our usual technique has been either to take deep bites with large sutures through each lip of the erosions and then through the valve sewing ring or to use Teflon strips to buttress the closure of the erosion and incorporate these sutures in the valve ring. Solid mooring of the sutures in this condition is essential; this may involve deep bites into the mitral valve or into the septum, and occasionally the conduction system must be sacrificed knowingly in order to accomplish a secure valve implantation.

Surgical Anatomy

The anatomy of the aortic valve is shown in Figures 14-3 and 14-4. Figure 14-3 shows the valve from above, with the orientation as usually seen through a standard transverse aortotomy.

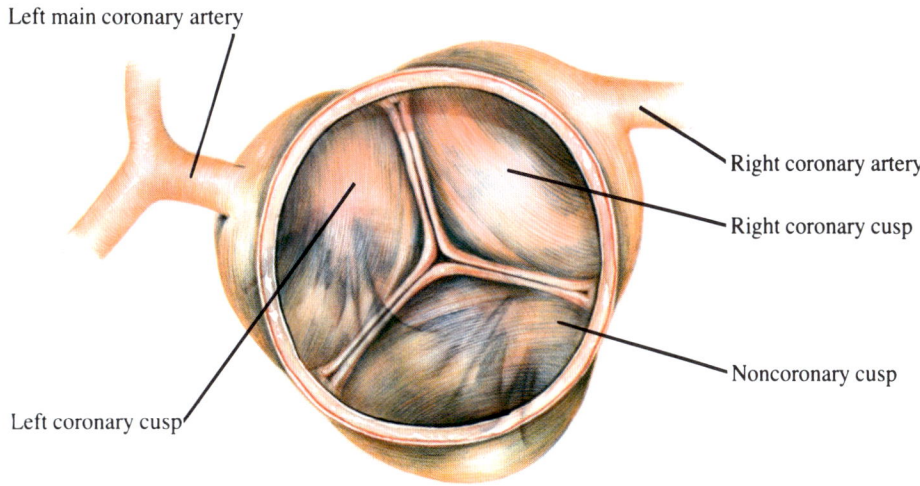

FIGURE 14-3

Aortic Valve Surgery

Figure 14-4 is an opened-out view of the aortic valve to illustrate the subvalvular anatomy. With the exception of the nomenclature of the cusps, the nomenclature is that of McAlpine.[74] Because the left ventricle has a common inlet and outlet, the anatomy of the aortic valve and mitral valve is intimately related.

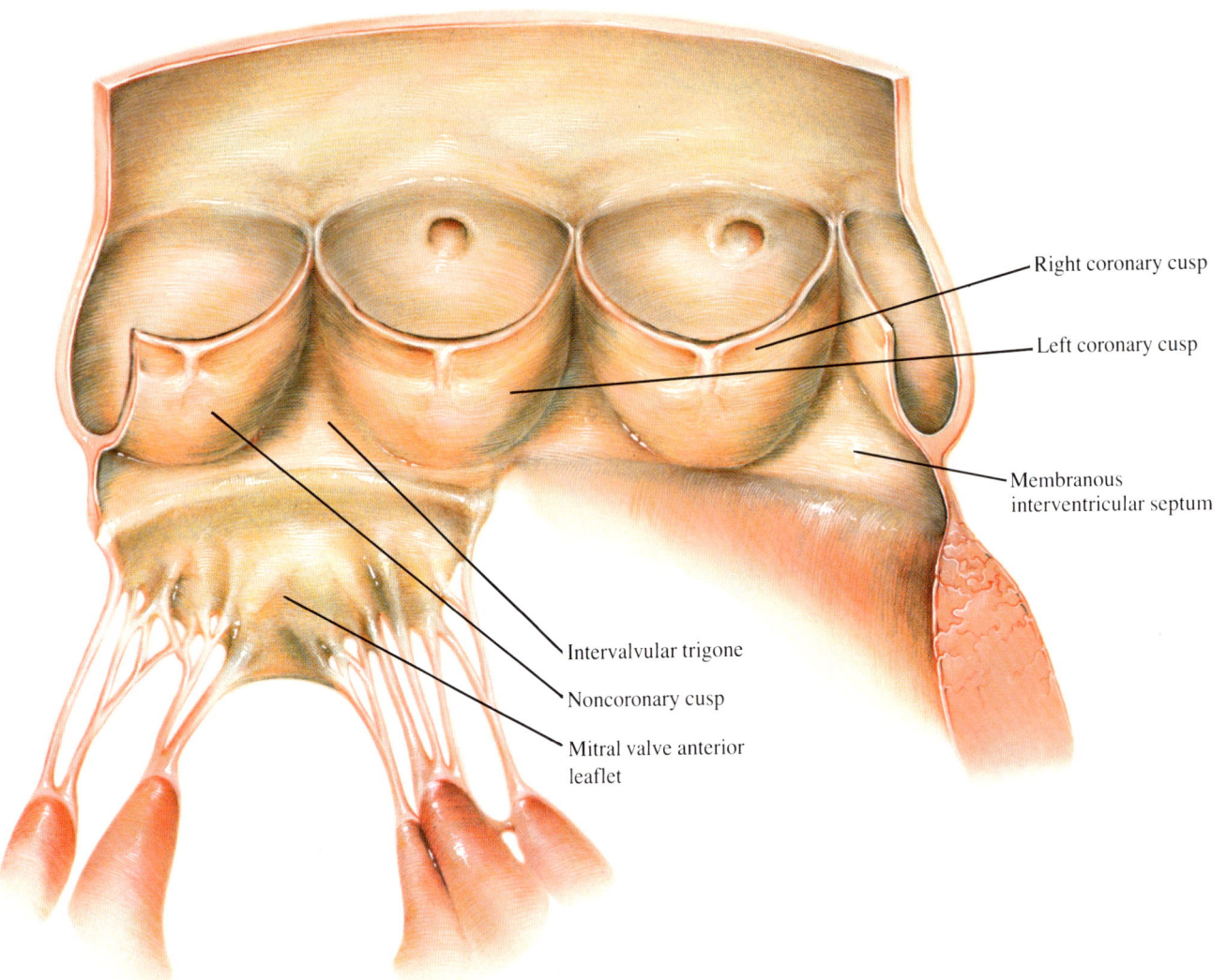

FIGURE 14-4

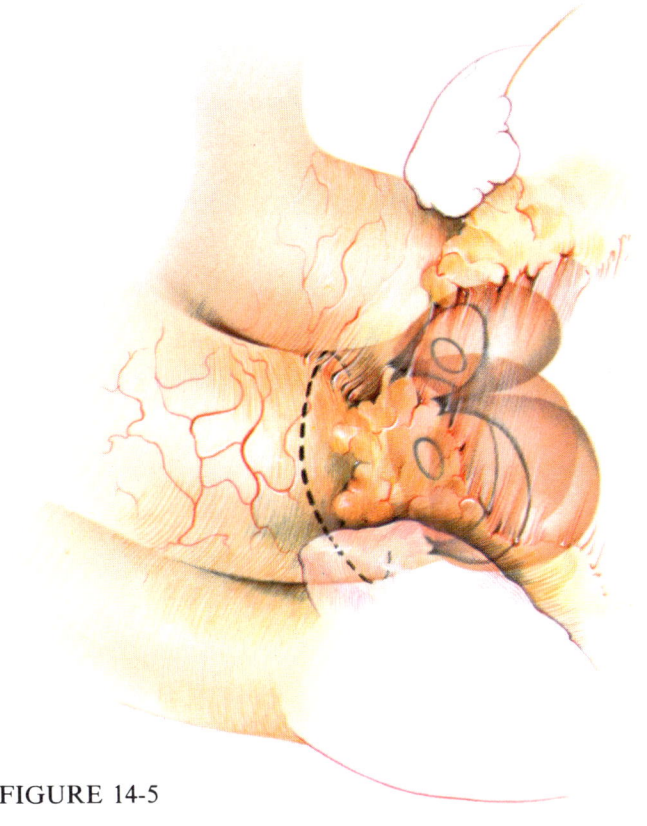

FIGURE 14-5

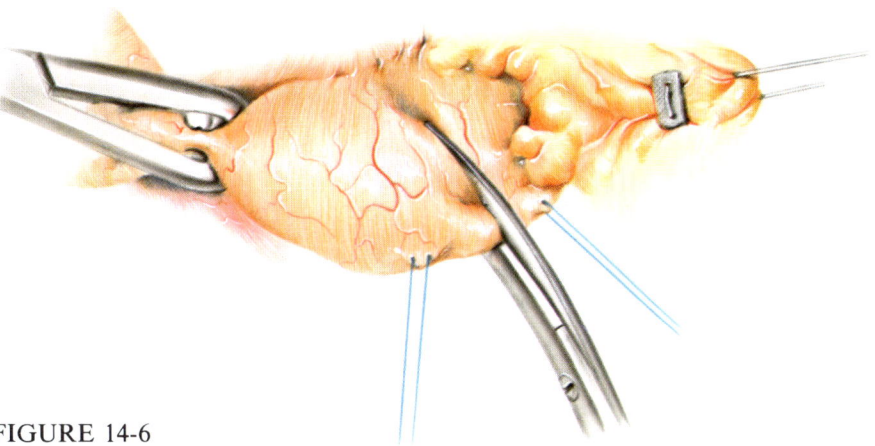

FIGURE 14-6

Technique

A transverse aortotomy is made (Figs. 14-5, 14-6). The incision should be made approximately 15 mm above the level of the right coronary artery. The incision should not be too low, since this can jeopardize the right coronary artery and create technical difficulties in valve seating and aortotomy closure. Erring on the high side is of little consequence, since the aortotomy can quickly be angled downward, and the anterior "lip" created by a high incision can be easily retracted. The aortotomy should be extended to approximately 10 mm above the commissure between the left coronary cusp and right coronary cusp and to a similar distance above the commissure between the left coronary cusp and the noncoronary cusp. Cold cardioplegic solution is injected into the coronary ostia via hand-held cannulas.

Retractors are placed, the valve is exposed (Fig. 14-7), and a strategy for excision is determined. The goal of excision is to establish a bed as free of calcium as is consistent with avoidance of injury to the aortic wall and the bundle of His. Many heavily calcified valves have calcification that stops prior to the anulus, leaving a thin zone of noncalcified attachment. In these instances, advantage may be taken of this morphologic feature by starting the incision with a scalpel in the calcium-free area near the anulus. This incision increases leaflet mobility, allowing more light under the leaflet, and more clearly indicates the area of subsequent incision. The incision can be completed with scissors.

If the valve does not contain a clear zone for incision, excision can be started with heavy scissors (Fig. 14-8). Incision is *not* made close to the anulus since such heavy calcification can obscure landmarks and a portion of the anulus can be inadvertently excised.

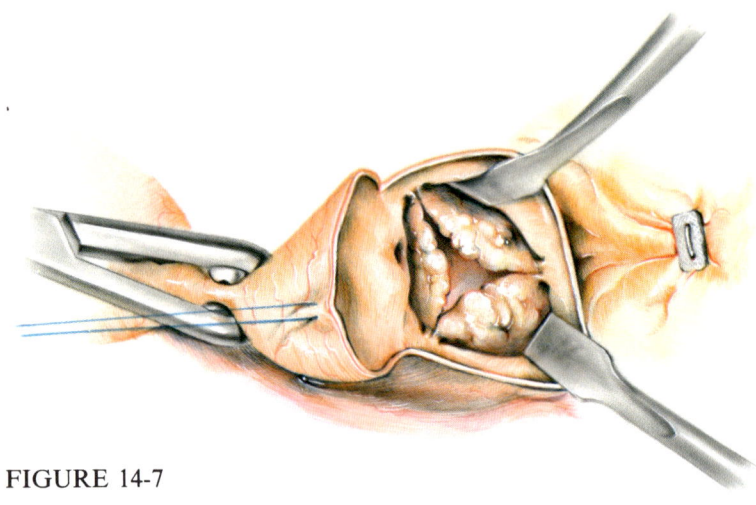

FIGURE 14-7

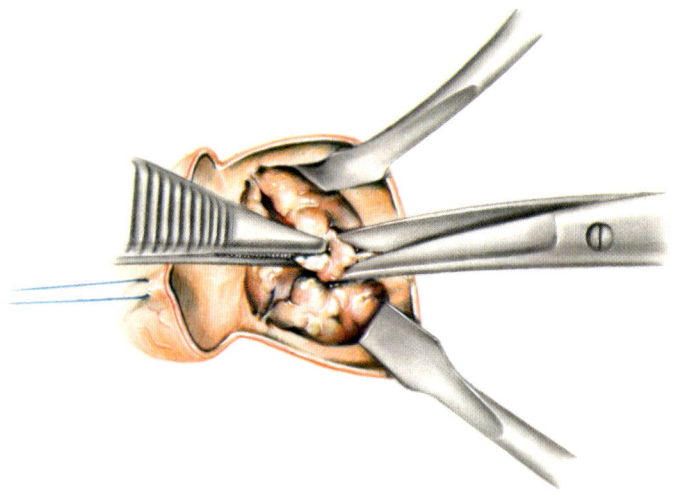

FIGURE 14-8

Debridement of the calcium is then performed with rongeurs (Fig. 14-9). The top is removed from the wall sucker to provide a vacuuming instrument to suction small fragments of calcium if they break off. The calcium can be crushed with the rongeur and then teased or peeled away from the anulus. Again, it is important to proceed cautiously to prevent removal of any of the anulus.

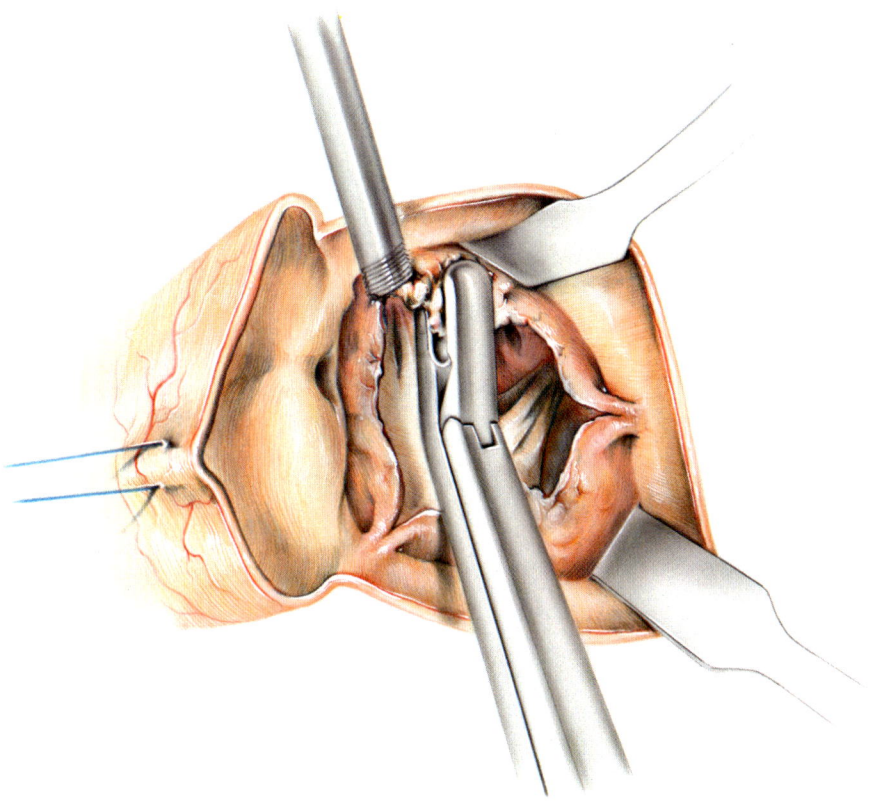

FIGURE 14-9

Calcification will sometimes extend down onto the base of the anterior leaflet of the mitral valve. A plane can usually be located between the calcium and the leaflet, and the calcium peeled off (Fig. 14-10). The debrided anulus is flexible, accepts sutures easily, and coapts to the valve ring tightly and completely.

Sutures of either 3-0 or 2-0 Teflon-coated Dacron are placed near each commissure for retraction (Fig. 14-11). These sutures will also be prosthesis sutures. They may be placed during debridement as needed for retraction and exposure.

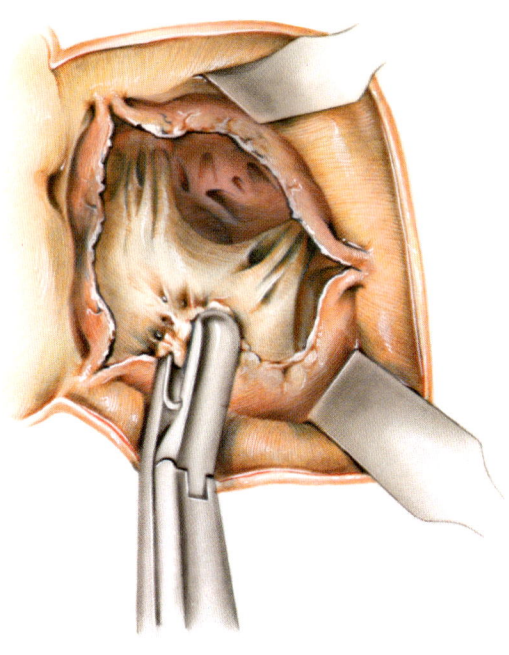

FIGURE 14-10

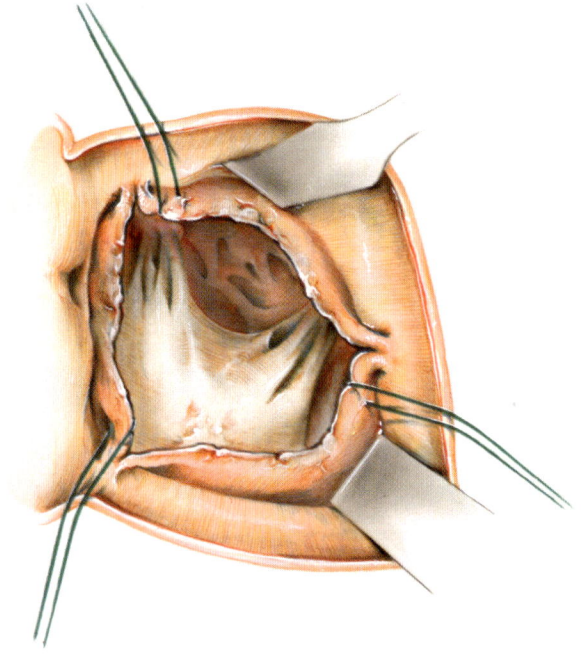

FIGURE 14-11

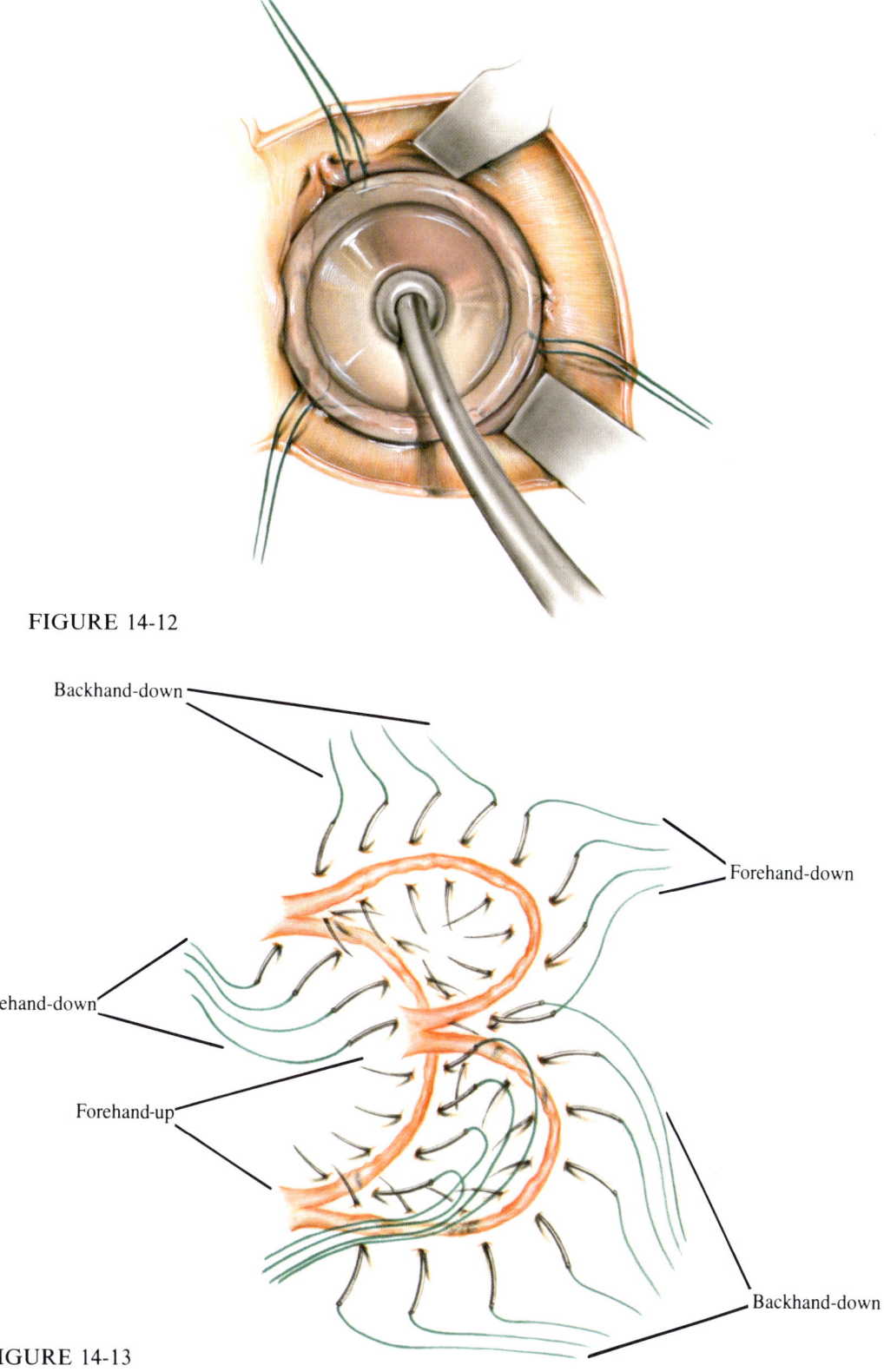

FIGURE 14-12

FIGURE 14-13

The anulus is then sized (Fig. 14-12). Progressively larger sizers are used. The proper fit for a Starr-Edwards valve is shown in Figure 14-12. Whatever valve is used, the valve should sit *in* the anulus, not *on* the anulus. Trying to "stuff in" a valve that is too large can cause disaster, such as coronary ostial impingement or tearing of the anulus.

The standard sutures for aortic valve replacement are shown in Figure 14-13. The sutures are started on the left coronary cusp near the commissure

Aortic Valve Surgery

with the noncoronary cusp, with forehand-up sutures (Fig. 14-14). The sutures may then be placed directly in the valve sewing ring or they may be clamped and held (Fig. 14-15) for later placement in the valve. Retraction of the sutures toward the patient's right facilitates exposure of the cusp.

As the left coronary cusp reaches its nadir and begins to come up to the commissure with the right coronary cusp, the easiest suture is usually a forehand-down (Fig. 14-16), either with the elbow in tight toward the body or with the elbow across the table.

The beginning sutures in the right coronary cusp are backhand-down with the elbow out (Fig. 14-17). As the cusp rises from its deepest point, forehand sutures are taken (Fig. 14-18).

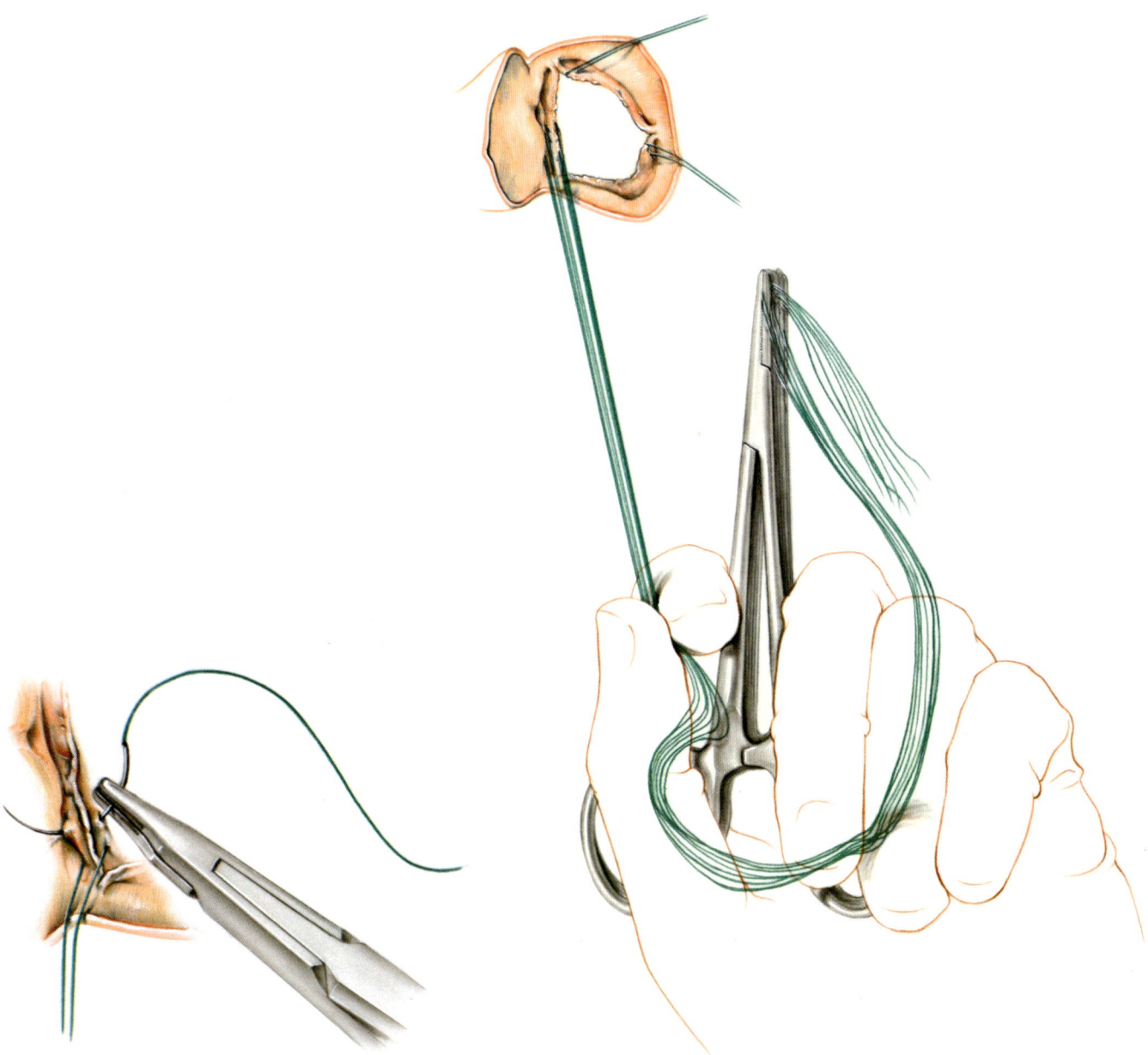

FIGURE 14-14

FIGURE 14-15

Replacement

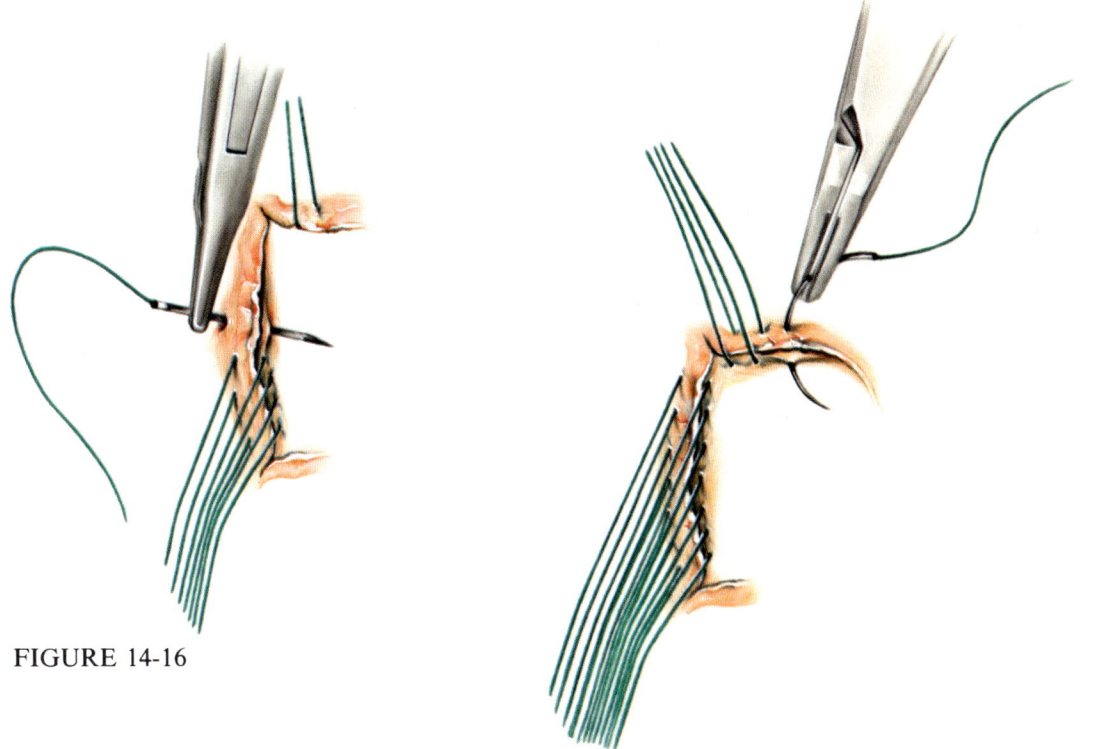

FIGURE 14-16

FIGURE 14-17

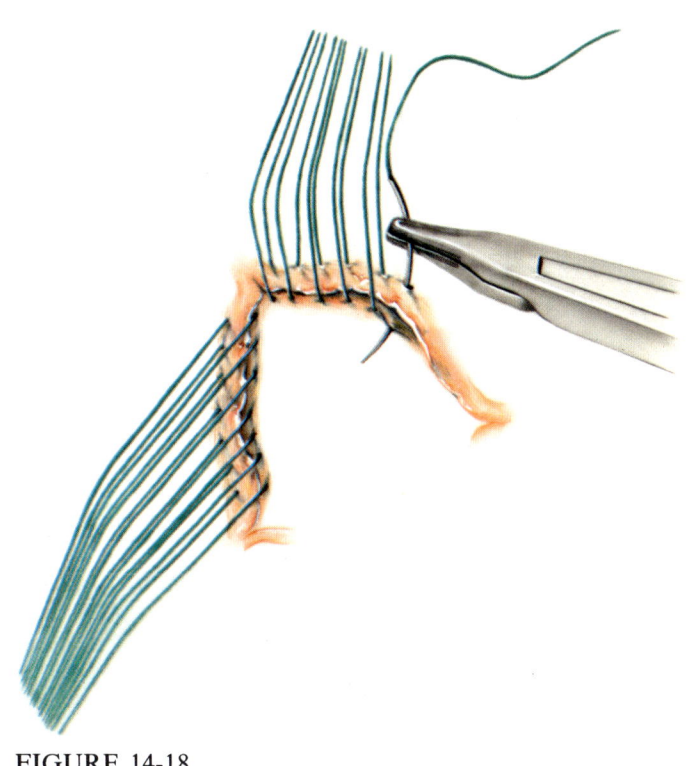

FIGURE 14-18

221

Aortic Valve Surgery

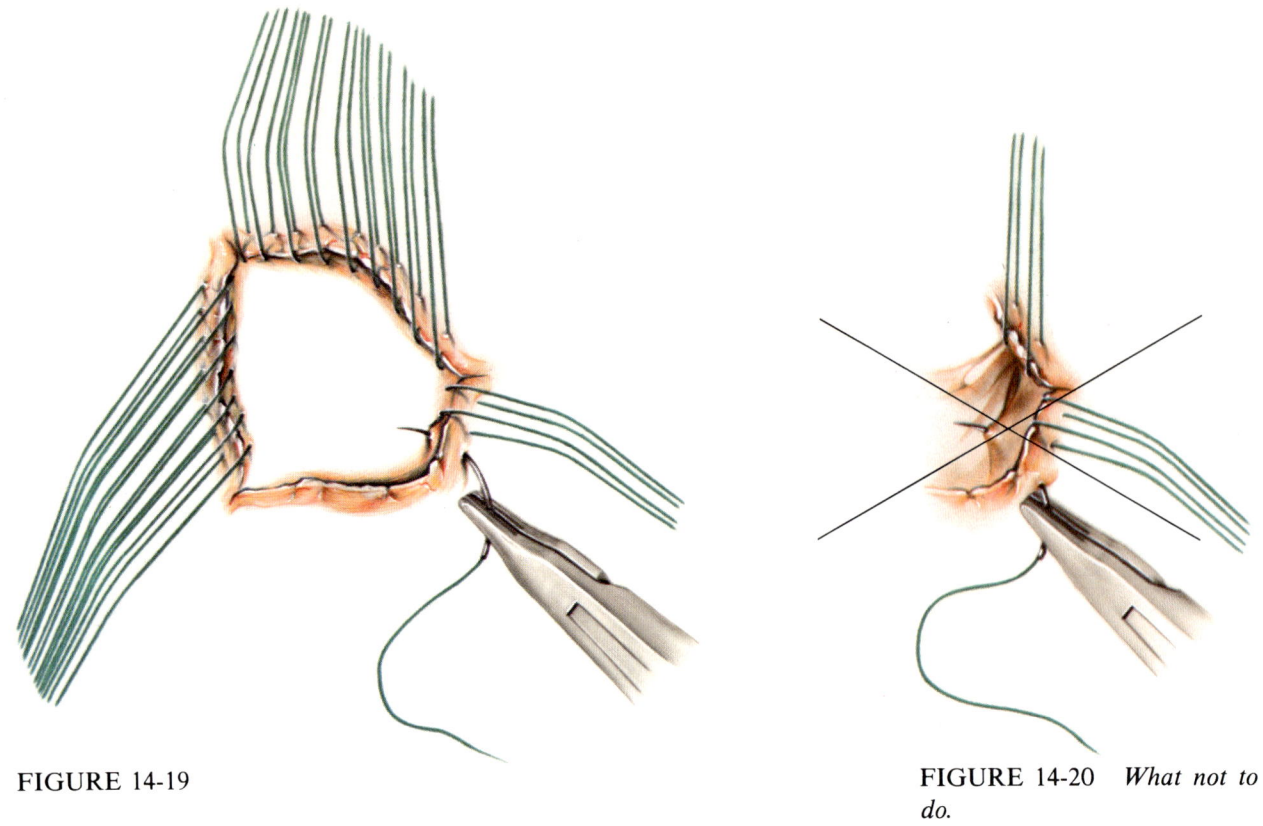

FIGURE 14-19

FIGURE 14-20 *What not to do.*

The noncoronary cusp is sutured backhand-down (Fig. 14-19). Underneath the commissure with the right coronary cusp is the membranous septum. A deep suture in this area *should not* be taken (Fig. 14-20), since such a suture can injure the conduction system. Retraction of the noncoronary cusp sutures toward the patient's right groin facilitates exposure.

Sutures are placed in the sewing ring in a vertical mattress fashion, with the suture coming out the ventricular side taking a broad bite through the sewing ring, and the suture on the aortic side taking a smaller bite in the lip (Fig. 14-21). This technique pulls the anulus into the compressible ring as the sutures are tied, for good sewing ring–anulus coaptation. The sutures are tied with slight compression of the sewing ring (Fig. 14-22).

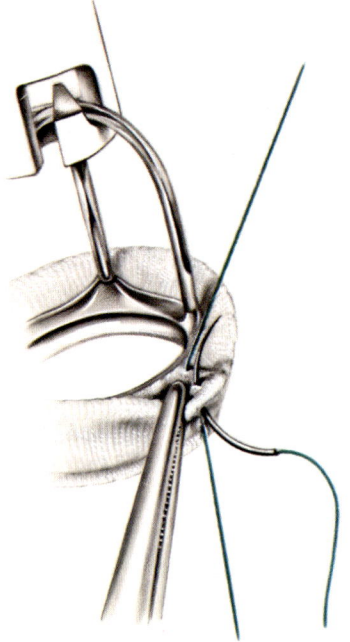

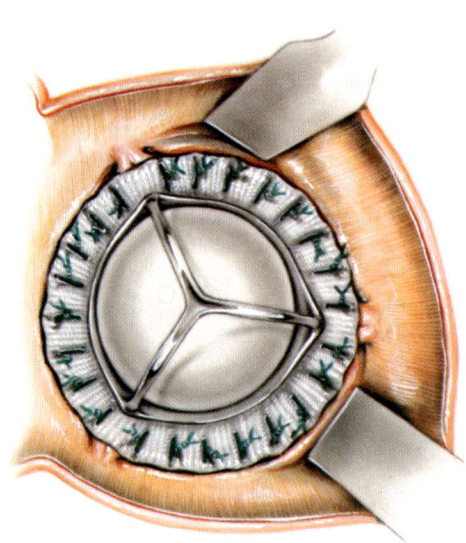

FIGURE 14-21

FIGURE 14-22

Anular Enlargement
The aortotomy is extended through the commissure between the left coronary cusp and the noncoronary cusp, onto the mitral valve for 10–15 mm (Fig. 14-23). The left atrium is not usually entered. A woven Dacron graft is then sewn to the mitral leaflet, across the incised anulus, and up onto the aortotomy (Fig. 14-24). The valve is placed at the normal anular level. At the area of the patch, horizontal mattress sutures are taken through the valve ring, brought through the patch, and tied over Teflon pledgets. The patch is carried up and incorporated in the aortotomy closure (Fig. 14-25).

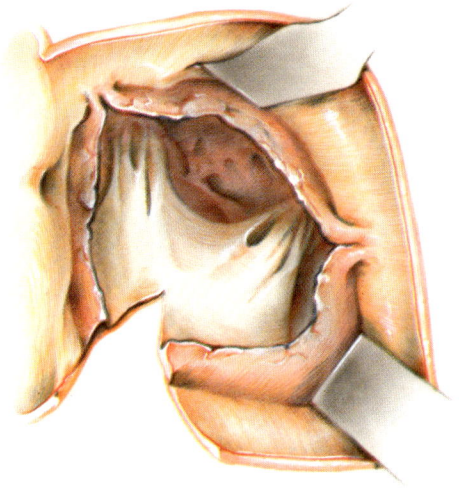

FIGURE 14-23

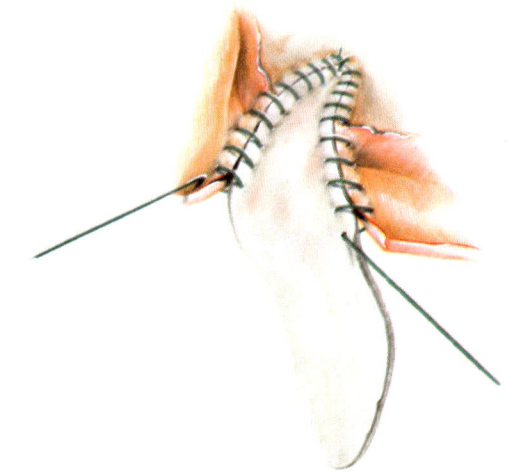

FIGURE 14-24

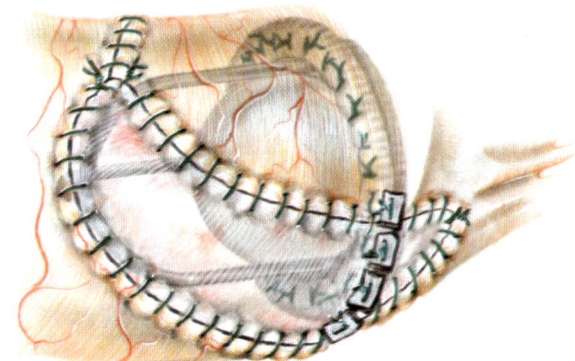

FIGURE 14-25

Results

Operative Mortality
Isolated aortic valve replacement can be performed with an operative mortality of 0%–2%.[1,46,103] Similarly excellent results can be achieved with combined valve replacement and coronary artery bypass.[96] Valve replacement earlier in the course of disease and improving techniques of myocardial protection are both likely to lower the overall risk of aortic valve replacement.

Ventricular Function
Aortic stenosis: Successful, uncomplicated valve replacement results in maintenance of ejection fraction that is normal preoperatively.[59,84,85,115] In addition, left ventricular mass decreases, and mean velocity of fiber shortening increases.[84] Marked reversal of impaired left ventricular function usually occurs.[20,30,109] Smith and co-workers[109] reported ten patients with an increase of mean ejection fraction from 34% to 63%. Croke and colleagues[30] reported seven patients with an increase in average ejection fraction from 13% to 45%. Ejection fractions improve in all patients in congestive heart failure if there is no perioperative myocardial infarction.[109]

The reversibility of impaired ventricular function may occur because the impaired cardiac performance preoperatively is due to inappropriately high wall stress—"afterload mismatch"—rather than depressed contractility.[20,48,99] Fifer and colleagues[35] have shown that contractile function, as characterized by the isovolumic rate of stress development, is not necessarily impaired in chronic pressure-overload hypertrophy. The rate of stress development was nearly identical in patients with aortic stenosis and in normal subjects. Gunther and co-workers[48] have shown that left ventricular wall thickness and geometry are closely correlated with ventricular performance in patients with pressure-overload hypertrophy due to aortic stenosis. They suggest that poor cardiac performance may often be due to inadequate hypertrophy (or inappropriate geometry) rather than to depression of myocardial contractility.

Aortic regurgitation: As in aortic stenosis, ejection fraction that is normal preoperatively remains normal.[59,84,115] Unfortunately, impaired ventricular function does not always improve. Clark and colleagues[22] reported a series of patients with an average preoperative left ventricular ejection fraction of 0.43. Left ventricular systolic pump function improved in only 50% of patients. Regardless of preoperative systolic pump function, successful valve replacement usually results in decreases in left ventricular mass, diastolic and systolic volumes, and end-diastolic pressure.[22,84]

Late Survival
The major determinant of late survival after aortic valve replacement is preoperative left ventricular function.[10,11,49,53,102,106,109] Large series of patients, with varied valvular pathology and type of prosthesis, have shown five-year survival (excluding operative death) of approximately 75%–85%, and this survival is for ball valves, tilting-disc valves, and porcine heterografts.[6,68,69,83,112] The majority of late deaths are not caused by prosthesis-related complications, but by myocardial factors—emphasizing again that the most critical factor relating to the success of valvular surgery is the functional and structural status of the myocardium preoperatively. Greves and colleagues,[46] from the University of Oregon, reported early and late survival for patients undergoing aortic valve replacement for severe, isolated aortic regurgitation from 1973 to 1978. In patients with ejection fractions over 0.50, there were no operative deaths and no late deaths at an average follow-up of five years.

Prosthesis Hemodynamics
All three types of prosthesis have similar hemodynamics in the commonly used sizes (23–25 mm). There is usually a small resting transvalvular gradient of 10–20 mm Hg, which increases to 20–30 mm Hg with exercise.[16,56,104]

Prosthesis-Related Complications (Table 14-1)
Thromboembolism: The rate of thromboembolism for the ball valve is 3.3%/patient-year[68,69] and for the tilting-disc valve is 0.5%/patient-year,[6,118] in patients maintained on continuous anticoagulation. Some reports of remarkably low thromboembolic rates (0.0%/patient-year) for the tilting-disc valve have appeared.[118] Approximately half of the thromboembolic episodes are minor—there is no residual neurologic deficit or peripheral or coronary embolic complications. The Bjork-Shiley tilting-disc valve has the potentially catastrophic complication of prosthetic thrombosis, occurring at a rate of about 0.3%/patient-year.[6] This complication may be reduced by the new convexoconcave disc.[6]

Overall, thromboembolism rates for the porcine heterografts are disappointingly similar to those found with mechanical prostheses: approximately 1.2%/patient-year.[23,83] However, most patients with porcine valves do not require continuous anticoagulation and therefore are not exposed to its risk.

Anticoagulant-related morbidity and mortality: Patients on continuous anticoagulation have a constant and continuing risk of hemorrhagic complications. The probability of a major hemorrhage is approximately 1.5%/patient-year, and the risk of minor bleeding is about the same.[54] The risk of fatal hemorrhage is approximately 0.1%/patient-year in our experience.

Structural failure: Structural failure has not occurred with the noncloth-covered (Silastic ball) prosthesis.[69] No structural failures have occurred in large series of Bjork-Shiley tilting-disc prostheses.[6] Structural failure is also rare in porcine prostheses followed to five years.[23,83]

However, the intrinsic weakness and vulnerability of tissue mandate continuous assessment of durability of bioprostheses. Ultrastructural evaluation of porcine xenograft valves after implantation has shown changes that are proportional to the duration of implantation.[34] As mentioned in Chapter 10, these changes include progressive collagen disruption, erosion of the valve surfaces, accumulation of lipid, and formation of platelet aggregates. The relationship of these changes to long-term durability is as yet undetermined. Well-founded conclusions regarding durability of porcine xenograft valves will require follow-up well into the 1980s. The most likely projection is that the porcine xenograft, as currently fabricated, is a ten-year valve.[78]

TABLE 14-1. A Comparison of Current Aortic Valve Prostheses

	Caged-ball[68*,69*] (Starr-Edwards 1200/60 & 2400)	Tilting-disc[6,118] (Bjork-Shiley)	Tissue[23,83] (Hancock xenograft)
Operative survivors	449	376	739
Total years of follow-up	992	1318	1710
(mean, maximum)	(2.2, 7)	(3.5, 10)	(2.3, 6)
Structural failures (%/patient-yr)	0	0	0.2(±0.1)
Prosthetic thrombosis (%/patient-yr)	0.1(±0.1)	0.3(±0.1)	0.2(±0.1)
Thromboembolism (%/patient-yr)	3.3(±0.6)	0.5(±0.2)	1.2(±0.3)

* Using recent time-frame only (data from patients who had valves implanted since 1973).

Surgical Relief of Other Forms of Left Ventricular Outflow Obstruction

Supravalvular Stenosis
Supravalvular aortic stenosis is a rare condition. The most common anatomy is narrowing just above the commissures.[94] Surgical treatment has consisted of patch enlargement into the noncoronary sinus.[76,94,111] Patch enlargement by incision into the right and noncoronary sinuses has also been recommended.[32] In the case of diffuse narrowing of the ascending aorta, creation of a left ventricle-to-aorta conduit is frequently the best treatment.[28]

Subaortic Membrane
Membranous subvalvular aortic stenosis is usually caused by a discrete membrane immediately beneath and unattached to the aortic valve.[57,58,80] It is usually circumferential and has continuity with the anterior leaflet of the mitral valve.

Surgical excision is straightforward, providing the bases of the aortic leaflets are not attached to the membranous ring. The aortic valve cusps are retracted and the membrane grasped and retracted posteriorly. The initial incision is made anteriorly under the right coronary cusp with a sharp-pointed blade. The incision is carried clockwise with careful assessment of the contiguous structures. Particular care is necessary near the bundle of His and the anterior leaflet of the mitral valve. The membrane can frequently be excised in one piece. In the case of extreme septal muscular hypertrophy, a myotomy may be added to ensure adequate relief of obstruction.

Idiopathic Hypertrophic Subaortic Stenosis
Idiopathic hypertrophic subaortic stenosis (IHSS) presents a broad spectrum of anatomy, physiology, and clinical course.[15,52,72] The treatment of IHSS is primarily medical.[38] Patients with large resting or provoked gradients are candidates for surgical therapy.[79]

Several operations have been proposed for treatment of IHSS, including (1) left ventriculomyotomy and myectomy through the aortic valve,[79,114] (2) myectomy with a combined approach through the aorta and left ventricle,[2] (3) septal myectomy via right ventriculotomy,[25] and (4) mitral valve replacement.[26] Our surgical procedure of choice is transaortic myectomy as described by Morrow.[79] This operation results in long-lasting clinical improvement in most patients.[73]

References

1. Adams PX, Cunningham JN, Trehan NK, Brazier JR, Reed GE, Spencer FC: Clinical experience using potassium-induced cardioplegia with hypothermia in aortic valve replacement. J Thorac Cardiovasc Surg 75:564, 1978.
2. Agnew TM, Barratt-Boyes BG, Brandt PWT, Roche AHG, Lowe JB, O'Brien KP: Surgical resection in idiopathic hypertrophic subaortic stenosis with a combined approach through aorta and left ventricle. J Thorac Cardiovasc Surg 74:307, 1977.
3. Anderson RP, Bonchek LI, Wood JA, Chapman RP, Starr A: The safety of combined aortic valve replacement and coronary bypass grafting. Ann Thorac Surg 15:249, 1973.
4. Barnhorst DA, Oxman HA, Connolly DC, Pluth JR, Danielson GK, Wallace RB, McGoon DC: Long-term follow-up of isolated replacement of the aortic or mitral valve with the Starr-Edwards prosthesis. Am J Cardiol 35:228, 1975.
5. Bernhard WF, Keane JF, Fellows KE, Litwin SB, Gross RE: Progress and

problems in the surgical management of congenital aortic stenosis. J Thorac Cardiovasc Surg 66:404, 1973.
6. Bjork VO, Henze A: Ten years' experience with the Bjork-Shiley tilting disc valve. J Thorac Cardiovasc Surg 78:331, 1979.
7. Blank RH, Pupello DF, Bessone LN, Harrison EE, Sbar S: Method of managing the small aortic annulus during valve replacement. Ann Thorac Surg 22:356, 1976.
8. Bolen JL, Holloway EL, Zener JC, Harrison DC, Alderman EL: Evaluation of left ventricular function in patients with aortic regurgitation using afterload stress. Circulation 53:132, 1976.
9. Bonchek LI, Anderson RP, Rosch J: Should coronary arteriography be performed routinely before valve replacement? Am J Cardiol 31:462, 1973.
10. Bonchek LI, Starr A: Ball valve prostheses: Current appraisal of late results. Am J Cardiol 35:843, 1975.
11. Bonow RO, Henry WL, Kent KM, Ware JW, Glancy DL, Redwood DR, Itscoitz SB, McIntosh CL, Conkle DM, Morrow AG, Epstein SE: Predictors of late death due to congestive heart failure following operation for aortic regurgitation (abstr). Am J Cardiol 41:382, 1978.
12. Borer JS, Bacharach SL, Green MV, Kent KM, Henry WL, Rosing DR, Seides SF, Johnston GS, Epstein SE: Exercise-induced left ventricular dysfunction in symptomatic and asymptomatic patients with aortic regurgitation: assessment with radionuclide cineangiography. Am J Cardiol 42:351, 1978.
13. Borer JS, Rosing DR, Kent KM, Bacharach SL, Green MV, McIntosh CJ, Morrow AG, Epstein SE: Left ventricular function at rest and during exercise after aortic valve replacement in patients with aortic regurgitation. Am J Cardiol 44:1297, 1979.
14. Boyd AD, Spencer FC, Isom W, Cunningham JN, Reed GE, Acinapura AJ, Tice DA: Infective endocarditis: an analysis of 54 surgically treated patients. J Thorac Cardiovasc Surg 73:23, 1977.
15. Braunwald E, Lambrew CT, Rockoff SD, Ross J Jr, Morrow AG: Idiopathic hypertrophic subaortic stenosis: I. A description of the disease based upon an analysis of 64 patients. Circulation 30:3, 1964.
16. Bristow JD, Kremkau EL: Hemodynamic changes after valve replacement with Starr-Edwards prostheses. Am J Cardiol 35:716, 1975.
17. Bristow JD, McCord CW, Starr A, Ritzmann LW, Griswold HE: Clinical and hemodynamic results of aortic valvular replacement with a ball valve prosthesis. Circulation 29:36, 1964.
18. Bristow JD, Parker BM, Haug WA: Hemopericardium following rupture of a bacterial aortic sinus aneurysm. Am J Cardiol 6:355, 1960.
19. Buckley MJ, Mundth ED, Daggett WM, Austen WG: Surgical management of the complications of sepsis involving the aortic valve, aortic root, and ascending aorta. Ann Thorac Surg 12:391, 1971.
20. Carabello BA, Green LH, Grossman W, Cohn LH, Koster JK, Collins JJ: Hemodynamic determinants of prognosis of aortic valve replacement in critical aortic stenosis and advanced congestive heart failure. Circulation 62:42, 1980.
21. Chesler E, Korns ME, Porter GE, Reyes CN, Edwards JE: False aneurysm of the left ventricle secondary to bacterial endocarditis with perforation of the mitral-aortic intervalvular fibrosa. Circulation 37:518, 1968.
22. Clark DG, McAnulty JH, Rahimtoola SH: Valve replacement in aortic insufficiency with left ventricular dysfunction. Circulation 61:411, 1980.
23. Cohn LH, Koster JK, Mee RBB, Collins JJ: Long-term follow-up of the Hancock bioprosthetic heart valve. Circulation 60(Suppl I):I-87, 1979.
24. Conkle DM, Jones M, Morrow AG: Treatment of congenital aortic stenosis. Arch Surg 107:649, 1973.
25. Cooley DA, Bloodwell RD, Hallman GL, LaSorte AF, Leachman RD, Chapman DW: Surgical treatment of muscular subaortic stenosis: results from septectomy in twenty-six patients. Circulation 35,36(Suppl I):I-124, 1967.
26. Cooley DA, Leachman RD, Hallman GL, Gerami S, Hall RJ: Idiopathic hyper-

trophic subaortic stenosis: surgical treatment including mitral valve replacement. Arch Surg 103:606, 1971.
27. Cooley DA, Norman JC: Techniques in Cardiac Surgery. Houston, Texas Medical Press, 1975, p 130.
28. Cooley DA, Norman JC, Mullins CE, Grace RR: Left ventricle to abdominal aorta conduits for relief of aortic stenosis. Cardiovasc Dis, Bull Texas Heart Inst 2:376, 1975.
29. Copeland JG, Griepp RB, Stinson EB, Shumway NE: Long-term follow-up after isolated aortic valve replacement. J Thorac Cardiovasc Surg 74:875, 1977.
30. Croke RP, Pifarre R, Sullivan H, Gunnar R, Loeb H: Reversal of advanced left ventricular dysfunction following aortic valve replacement for aortic stenosis. Ann Thorac Surg 24:38, 1977.
31. Danielson GK, Titus JL, DuShane JW: Successful treatment of aortic valve endocarditis and aortic root abscesses by insertion of prosthetic valve in ascending aorta and placement of bypass grafts to coronary arteries. J Thorac Cardiovasc Surg 67:443, 1974.
32. Doty DB, Polansky DB, Jenson CB: Supravalvular aortic stenosis. Repair by extended aortoplasty. J Thorac Cardiovasc Surg 74:362, 1971.
33. Edmunds LH Jr, Wagner HR, Heymann MA: Aortic valvulotomy in neonates. Circulation 61:421, 1980.
34. Ferrans VJ, Spray TL, Billingham ME, Roberts WE: Structural changes in glutaraldehyde-treated porcine heterografts used as substitute cardiac valves. Am J Cardiol 41:1159, 1978.
35. Fifer MA, Gunther S, Grossman W, Mirsky I, Carabello B, Barry WH: Myocardial contractile function in aortic stenosis as determined from the rate of stress development during isovolumic systole. Am J Cardiol 44:1318, 1979.
36. Fischl SJ, Gorlin R, Herman MV: Cardiac shape and function in aortic valve disease: physiologic and clinical implications. Am J Cardiol 39:170, 1977.
37. Forman R, Firth BG, Barnard MS: Prognostic significance of preoperative left ventricular ejection fraction and valve lesion in patients with aortic valve replacement. Am J Cardiol 45:1120, 1980.
38. Frank MJ, Abdulla AM, Canedo MI, Saylors RE: Long-term medical management of hypertrophic obstructive cardiomyopathy. Am J Cardiol 42:993, 1978.
39. Frank S, Johnson A, Ross J Jr: Natural history of valvular aortic stenosis. Br Heart J 35:41, 1973.
40. Frantz PT, Murray GF, Wilcox BR: Surgical management of left ventricular-aortic discontinuity complicating bacterial endocarditis. Ann Thorac Surg 29:1, 1980.
41. Friedman WF, Pappelbaum SJ: Indications for hemodynamic evaluation and surgery in congenital aortic stenosis. Pediatr Clin North Am 18:1207, 1971.
42. Girardet RE, Wheat MW: Technique of aortic valve replacement. J Thorac Cardiovasc Surg 71:446, 1976.
43. Goldschlager N, Pfeifer J, Cohn K, Popper R, Selzer A: The natural history of aortic regurgitation. A clinical and hemodynamic study. Am J Med 54:577, 1973.
44. Gault JH, Covell JW, Braunwald E, Ross J: Left ventricular performance following correction of free aortic regurgitation. Circulation 42:773, 1970.
45. Gonzalez-Lavin L, Scappatura E, Lise M, Ross ND: Mycotic aneurysms of the aortic root: a complication of aortic valve endocarditis. Ann Thorac Surg 9:551, 1970.
46. Greves J, Clark D, Greenberg B, McAnulty J, Starr A, Rahimtoola S: Late survival after valve replacement for severe isolated aortic incompetence (abstr). Am J Cardiol 45:440, 1980.
47. Grossman W, Jones D, McLaurin LP: Wall stress and patterns of hypertrophy in the human left ventricle. J Clin Invest 56:56, 1975.
48. Gunther S, Grossman W: Determinants of ventricular function in pressure-overload hypertrophy in man. Circulation 59:679, 1979.
49. Henry WL, Bonow RO, Borer JS, Kent KM, Ware JH, Redwood DR, Itscoitz

SB, McIntosh CL, Morrow AG, Epstein SE: Evaluation of aortic valve replacement in patients with valvular aortic stenosis. Circulation 61:814, 1980.
50. Henry WL, Bonow RO, Borer JS, Ware JH, Kent KM, Redwood DR, McIntosh CL, Morrow AG, Epstein SE: Observations on the optimum time for operative intervention for aortic regurgitation: I. Evaluation of the results of aortic valve replacement in symptomatic patients. Circulation 61:471, 1980.
51. Henry WL, Bonow RO, Rosing DR, Epstein SE: Observations on the optimum time for operative intervention for aortic regurgitation: II. Serial echocardiographic evaluation of asymptomatic patients. Circulation 61:484, 1980.
52. Henry WL, Clark CE, Epstein SE: Asymmetric septal hypertrophy (ASH): the unifying link in the IHSS disease spectrum. Circulation 47:827, 1973.
53. Hirshfield JW, Epstein SE, Roberts AJ, Glancy DL, Morrow AG: Indices predicting long-term survival after valve replacement in patients with aortic regurgitation and patients with aortic stenosis. Circulation 50:1190, 1974.
54. Isom OW, Spencer FC, Glassman E, Teiko P, Boyd AD, Cunningham JN: Long-term results in 1,375 patients undergoing valve replacement with the Starr-Edwards cloth-covered composite-seat prostheses: a six-year appraisal. Ann Surg 186:310, 1977.
55. Jack WD II, Kelly DT: Long-term follow-up of valvulotomy for congenital aortic stenosis. Am J Cardiol 38:231, 1976.
56. Jones EL, Craver JM, Morris DC, King SB III, Douglas JS Jr, Franch RH, Hatcher CR Jr, Morgan EA: Hemodynamic and clinical evaluation of the Hancock xenograft bioprosthesis for aortic valve replacement (with emphasis on management of the small aortic root). J Thorac Cardiovasc Surg 75:300, 1978.
57. Katz NM, Buckley MJ, Liberthson RR: Discrete membranous subaortic stenosis. Circulation 56:1034, 1977.
58. Kelly DT, Wulfsberg E, Rowe RD: Discrete subaortic stenosis. Circulation 46:309, 1972.
59. Kennedy JW, Doces J, Stewart DK: Left ventricular function before and following aortic valve replacement. Circulation 56:944, 1977.
60. Kirklin JW, Pacifico AD: Surgery for acquired valvular heart disease. N Engl J Med 288:133, 194, 1973.
61. Konno S, Imai Y, Iida Y, Nakajima M, Tatsuno K: A new method for prosthetic valve replacement in congenital aortic stenosis associated with hypoplasia of the aortic ring. J Thorac Cardiovasc Surg 70:910, 1975.
62. Kouchoukos NT, Karp RB, Lell WA: Replacement of the ascending aorta and aortic valve with a composite graft: results in 25 patients. Ann Thorac Surg 24:140, 1977.
63. Lakier JB, Khaja F, Magilligan DJ Jr, Goldstein S: Porcine xenograft valves: long-term (60–89 month) follow-up. Circulation 62:313, 1980.
64. Lakier JB, Lewis AB, Heymann MA, Stanger P, Hoffman JIE, Rudolph AM: Isolated aortic stenosis in the neonate. Natural history and hemodynamic considerations. Circulation 50:801, 1974.
65. Lawson RM, Bonchek LI, Menashe V, Starr A: Late results of surgery for left ventricular outflow tract obstruction in children. J Thorac Cardiovasc Surg 71:334, 1976.
66. Lefrak EA, Starr A: Cardiac Valve Prostheses. New York, Appleton-Century-Crofts, 1979.
67. Linhart JW, Wheat MW: Myocardial dysfunction following aortic valve replacement: the significance of coronary artery disease. J Thorac Cardiovasc Surg 54:259, 1967.
68. Macmanus Q, Grunkemeier G, Housman L, Maloney C, Harlan BJ, Starr A: Early results with composite-strut caged-ball prostheses. Am J Cardiol 46:566, 1980.
69. Macmanus Q, Grunkemeier GL, Lambert LE, Teply JF, Harlan BJ, Starr A: Year of operation as a risk factor in the late results of valve replacement. J Thorac Cardiovasc Surg 80:834, 1980.
70. Manouguian S, Seybold-Epting W: Patch enlargement of the aortic valve ring

by extending the aortic incision into the anterior mitral leaflet. J Thorac Cardiovasc Surg 78:402, 1979.
71. Maron BJ, Ferrans VJ, Roberts WC: Myocardial ultrastructure in patients with chronic aortic valve disease. Am J Cardiol 35:725, 1975.
72. Maron BJ, Lipson LC, Roberts WC, Savage DD, Epstein SE: "Malignant" hypertrophic cardiomyopathy: identification of a subgroup of families with unusually frequent premature death. Am J Cardiol 41:1133, 1978.
73. Maron BJ, Merrill WH, Freier PA, Kent KM, Epstein SE, Morrow AG: Long-term clinical course and symptomatic status of patients after operation for hypertrophic subaortic stenosis. Circulation 57:1205, 1978.
74. McAlpine WA: Heart and Coronary Arteries. Berlin, Heidelberg, New York, Springer-Verlag, 1975.
75. McAnulty JH, Rahimtoola SH: Surgery for infective endocarditis. JAMA 242:77, 1979.
76. McGoon DC, Mankin HT, Vlad P, Kirklin JW: The surgical treatment of supravalvular aortic stenosis. J Thorac Cardiovasc Surg 41:125, 1961.
77. Mills J, Utley J, Abbott J: Heart failure in infective endocarditis: predisposing factors, course, and treatment. Chest 66:2, 1974.
78. Morrow AG: Personal communication. 1980.
79. Morrow AG, Reitz BA, Epstein SE, Henry WL, Conkle DM, Itscoitz SB, Redwood DR: Operative treatment in hypertrophic subaortic stenosis: techniques and the results of pre- and postoperative assessment in 83 patients. Circulation 52:88, 1975.
80. Newfeld EA, Muster AJ, Paul MH, Idriss FS, Riker WL: Discrete subvalvular aortic stenosis in childhood. Am J Cardiol 38:53, 1976.
81. Okies JE, Bradshaw MW, Williams TW: Valve replacement in bacterial endocarditis. Chest 63:898, 1973.
82. O'Rourke RA, Crawford MH: Timing of valve replacement in patients with chronic aortic regurgitation. Circulation 61:493, 1980.
83. Oyer PE, Stinson EB, Reitz BA, Miller DC, Rossiter SJ, Shumway NE: Long-term evaluation of the porcine xenograft bioprosthesis. J Thorac Cardiovasc Surg 78:343, 1979.
84. Pantely G, Morton M, Rahimtoola SH: Effects of successful, uncomplicated valve replacement on ventricular hypertrophy, volume, and performance in aortic stenosis and in aortic incompetence. J Thorac Cardiovasc Surg 75:383, 1978.
85. Parker FB, Thomas FD, Poirier RA, Markowitz AHM, Eich RH: Left ventricular function following aortic valve replacement. J Thorac Cardiovasc Surg 79:121, 1980.
86. Peterson CR, Herr R, Crisera RV, Starr A, Bristow JD, Griswold HE: The failure of hemodynamic improvement after valve replacement surgery: etiology, diagnosis, and treatment. Ann Int Med 66:1, 1967.
87. Pupello DF, Blank RH, Bessone LN, Harrison E, Sbar S: Surgical management of the small aortic annulus: hemodynamic evaluation. Chest 74:163, 1978.
88. Rahimtoola SH: Early valve replacement for preservation of ventricular function? Am J Cardiol 40:472, 1977.
89. Rahimtoola SH (ed): Infective Endocarditis. New York, Grune & Stratton, 1978.
90. Rahimtoola SH: The problem of valve prosthesis–patient mismatch. Circulation 58:20, 1978.
91. Rahimtoola SH: Valve replacement should *not* be performed in all asymptomatic patients with severe aortic incompetence. J Thorac Cardiovasc Surg 79:163, 1980.
92. Rapaport E: Natural history of aortic and mitral valve disease. Am J Cardiol 35:221, 1975.
93. Rastan H, Koncz J: Aortoventriculoplasty. J Thorac Cardiovasc Surg 71:920, 1976.
94. Rastelli GB, McGoon DC, Ongley PA, Mankin GT, Kirklin JW: Surgical treatment of supravalvular aortic stenosis. Report of 16 cases and review of the literature. J Thorac Cardiovasc Surg 51:873, 1966.

95. Richardson JV, Karp RB, Kirklin JW, Dismukes WE: Treatment of infective endocarditis: a 10-year comparative analysis. Circulation 58:589, 1978.
96. Richardson JV, Kouchoukos NT, Wright JO III, Karp RB: Combined aortic valve replacement and myocardial revascularization: results in 220 patients. Circulation 59:75, 1979.
97. Rigo P, Alderson PO, Robertson RM, Becker LC, Wagner HN: Measurement of aortic and mitral regurgitation by gated cardiac blook pool scans. Circulation 60:306, 1979.
98. Rittenhouse EA, Sauvage LR, Stamm SJ, Mansfield PB, Hall DG, Herndon PS: Radical enlargement of the aortic root and outflow tract to allow valve replacement. Ann Thorac Surg 27:367, 1979.
99. Ross J Jr: Afterload mismatch and preload reserve: a conceptual framework for the analysis of ventricular function. Prog Cardiovasc Dis 18:255, 1976.
100. Ross J Jr, Braunwald E: Aortic stenosis. Circulation 38(Suppl V):V-61, 1968.
101. Ross J Jr, Sonnenblick EH, Taylor RR, Spotnitz HM, Covell JW: Diastolic geometry and sarcomere lengths in the chronically dilated canine left ventricle. Circ Res 28:49, 1971.
102. Samuels DA, Cureman GD, Friedlich AL, Buckley, MU Austen WG: Valve replacement for aortic regurgitation: long-term follow-up with factors influencing the results. Circulation 60:647, 1979.
103. Sapsford RN, Blackstone EH, Kirklin JW, Karp RB, Kouchoukos NT, Pacifico AD, Roe CR, Bradley EL: Coronary perfusion versus cold ischemic arrest during aortic valve surgery: a randomized study. Circulation 49:1190, 1974.
104. Schwarz F, Flameng W, Langebartels F, Sesto M, Walter P, Schlepper M: Impaired left ventricular function in chronic aortic valve disease: survival and function after replacement by Bjork-Shiley prosthesis. Circulation 60:48, 1979.
105. Selzer A: Cardiac valve replacement: an unanswered question. Am J Cardiol 37:322, 1976.
106. Shean FC, Austen WG, Buckley MJ, Mundth ED, Scannell JG, Daggett WM: Survival after Starr-Edwards aortic valve replacement. Circulation 44:1, 1971.
107. Shumacker HB Jr: Aneurysms of the aortic sinuses of Valsalva due to bacterial endocarditis, with special reference to their operative management. J Thorac Cardiovasc Surg 63:896, 1972.
108. Slaughter L, Morris JE, Starr A: Prosthetic valvular endocarditis: a 12-year review. Circulation 47:1319, 1973.
109. Smith N, McAnulty JH, Rahimtoola SH: Severe aortic stenosis with impaired left ventricular function and clinical heart failure: results of valve replacement. Circulation 58:255, 1978.
110. Sorensen SG, Groves BM, O'Rourke RA, Chaudhuri T: Noninvasive quantitation of valvular regurgitation by gated radionuclide angiography. J Nucl Med 20:629, 1979.
111. Starr A, Dotter C, Griswold HE: Supravalvular aortic stenosis: diagnosis and treatment. J Thorac Cardiovasc Surg 81:134, 1961.
112. Starr A, Grunkemeier G, Lambert LE, Thomas DR, Sugimura S, Lefrak EA: Aortic valve replacement: a ten-year followup of noncloth-covered vs cloth-covered caged ball prosthesis. Circulation 56(Suppl II):II-133, 1977.
113. Stinson EB, Griepp RB, Vosti K, Copeland JG, Shumway NE: Operative treatment of active endocarditis. J Thorac Cardiovasc Surg 71:659, 1976.
114. Syracuse DC, Gaudiani VA, Kastl DG, Henry WL, Morrow AG: Intraoperative, intracardiac echocardiography during left ventriculotomy and myectomy for hypertrophic subaortic stenosis. Circulation 58(Suppl I):I-23, 1978.
115. Thompson R, Yacoub M, Ahmed M, Seabra-Gomes R, Rickards A, Towers M: Influence of preoperative left ventricular function on results of homograft replacement of the aortic valve for aortic stenosis. Am J Cardiol 43:929, 1979.
116. Tompsett R, Lubash GD: Aortic valve perforation in bacterial endocarditis. Circulation 23:662, 1961.
117. Utley JR: Annular erosion and pericarditis: complications of endocarditis of the aortic root. J Thorac Cardiovasc Surg 64:76, 1972.

118. Walter P, Schwarz F, Scheld H, Hehrlein FW: Eight years of experience with the Bjork-Shiley tilting disc valve prosthesis in 833 patients. Thorac Cardiovasc Surg 27:178, 1979.
119. Wigle ED, Labrosse CJ: Sudden, severe aortic insufficiency. Circulation 32:708, 1965.

Left Ventricular Aneurysm

15

Left ventricular aneurysm develops following myocardial infarction in 10%–38% of patients.[1,7,35] Since Cooley's report[8] in 1958 of resection utilizing cardiopulmonary bypass the operation has become an established treatment for ventricular aneurysm causing congestive heart failure, intractable ventricular arrhythmia, or systemic emboli; resection of aneurysm in conjunction with coronary artery bypass for angina is also common.

This chapter concerns treatment of "true" ventricular aneurysm, as differentiated from "false" aneurysm. "True" left ventricular aneurysm is a full-thickness scar of the wall of the ventricle, is discrete from the surrounding viable myocardium, and has paradoxical or outward motion during systole. "False" left ventricular aneurysm is a contained rupture of the left ventricle;[25] the rupture is contained by adhesions of epicardium and pericardium. "False" aneurysms or pseudoaneurysms typically expand and are at risk of rupture;[13,15,16] for this reason their existence is indication for surgical treatment. Diagnosis of pseudoaneurysm and differentiation from "true" aneurysm can often be made noninvasively by echocardiography[32] and radionuclide angiography.[5]

Ventricular aneurysm must also be differentiated from a large area of akinetic myocardium—an area of fibrosis interspersed with viable muscle. Excision of akinetic myocardium is generally not indicated. Excision is associated with high operative mortality, poor late survival, and little, if any, improvement in symptoms.[21,39]

Resection

All aneurysms are opened and repaired. Plication—inversion or eversion of the aneurysm without opening it—is not performed. Plication has the definite hazard of dislodging mural thrombus and for this reason is not done. Using the open technique, little, if any, of the wall of a small aneurysm may be resected, but inclusion of the wall in the repair excludes the aneurysm from the functioning ventricle.

Indications

Congestive Heart Failure
Left ventricular aneurysm affects ventricular function adversely in a number of ways:[20] (1) the area of scar does not participate in contraction, (2) the expansion of the aneurysm diminishes forward flow of blood and decreases

the rate of development of tension in the viable muscle, and (3) the oxygen supply-demand balance in the viable myocardium can be upset, causing ischemic dysfunction of the ventricle. This increased myocardial oxygen demand is caused by the increased wall tension necessary to generate adequate chamber pressure as the ventricle enlarges (Laplace relationship).

Congestive heart failure is a common indication for surgery, being the primary indication in 23%–50% of patients.[6,10] Although congestive heart failure usually develops months after infarction, development of aneurysm may cause congestive heart failure as early as three weeks after infarction.[3,43]

Absolute contraindications to aneurysm resection have not been conclusively established, but a subset of patients in whom operative mortality is high and symptomatic improvement unlikely can be identified. Operative mortality and functional result following aneurysmectomy are best predicted by the contraction of the residual ventricle.[2,6,19,22,28,40,45] Qualitative analysis of residual ventricular function has been described by Burton and co-workers.[6] They found an operative mortality of 9.8% and five-year survival of 80% in patients with "good" contraction of the residual ventricle, whereas patients with "poor" contraction had an operative mortality of 34% and a five-year survival of 36%.

Quantitative analyses of the function of the residual ventricle have been described, including basilar fractional area reduction, contractile segment ejection fraction, and basilar half ejection fraction.[19,22,45] Kapelanski and colleagues[19] found that patients undergoing urgent aneurysmectomy with a basilar half ejection fraction below 30% had an 89% mortality, whereas patients with a basilar half ejection fraction over 30% had only 18% mortality. Watson and colleagues[45] found high operative mortality and poor functional improvement in patients with a contractile ejection fraction below 44%. Patients with a contractile ejection fraction over 45% all survived and had marked functional improvement.

Continued study of residual ventricular function is likely to improve selection of patients for surgery. Radionuclide studies will be an important component of such evaluation.[4,12,14,31,42,46]

Angina Pectoris
In the early years of cardiac surgery, angina was an infrequent indication for aneurysm resection. With the development of coronary artery surgery, unsuspected aneurysms were diagnosed in patients undergoing evaluation of angina. The increasing number of aneurysms being diagnosed has markedly increased the incidence of angina as a primary or associated indication for surgery. In a recent report from the Cleveland Clinic,[10] angina alone or angina with congestive heart failure was the indication for surgery in 63% of patients. Aneurysms discovered incidentally in the study of patients with angina pectoris should be resected in conjunction with the performance of coronary artery surgery.

Ventricular Arrhythmia
Ventricular aneurysms can be associated with serious ventricular arrhythmias. Medical management may not be successful in the management of these arrhythmias. Intractable ventricular arrhythmia as the primary indication for surgery ranges from 8% to 27%.[6,10,33] Ventricular aneurysmectomy, however, is not always effective in controlling the arrhythmia, with failure rates approaching 50%.[6,10] The development of operative mapping and endocardial excision[18] or encircling endocardial ventriculotomy[17] in association with aneurysmectomy holds promise of improving the results of surgery for arrhythmia, as may the use of implantable ventricular defibrillators.[26]

Systemic Embolism
Mural thrombi are commonly associated with ventricular aneurysms, found in approximately 60%.[6,11,38] However, systemic emboli are rare, and systemic embolism is the least frequent indication for surgery, accounting for only 2%–5% of patients.[6,10,23] It does not appear that chronic anticoagulation has any effect on the frequency of preoperative systemic arterial embolization or the prevalence of left ventricular mural thrombus found at surgery.[38]

Surgical Strategy

Myocardial Preservation
Cold potassium crystalloid cardioplegia is the usual method of myocardial preservation (Chapter 6). Ischemic arrest at moderate hypothermia may also be used if the time of aneurysm repair is less than 15 minutes.

Management of Coexistent Conditions
Coronary artery disease: All patients undergoing study of ventricular aneurysm should also undergo coronary arteriography. We perform saphenous vein bypass to vessels with 50% or more narrowing of luminal diameter and satisfactory distal vessels. Bypass is performed even if angina is not present. Our rationale for this practice is the strong suggestion that coexistent coronary artery surgery does not increase operative mortality,[10,37] may decrease operative mortality,[10] and appears to improve survival.[10,33] Patients who have had complete revascularization for multiple-vessel disease in association with aneurysmectomy have the same survival at seven years as those patients who have only single-vessel disease to the area of aneurysm.[10]

Distal anastomoses are usually performed after resection of the aneurysm. Proximal anastomoses are performed over a partial occluding clamp while the vented, beating, nonworking heart recovers from the period of cardioplegic arrest.

Mitral regurgitation: Mitral valve replacement may be performed through the open aneurysm from the left ventricular side[9] or through the standard left atriotomy.

Ventricular septal defect: The defect in the ventricular septum is closed in the standard fashion (Chapter 16) through the open aneurysm.

Surgical Anatomy
The vast majority of left ventricular aneurysms (approximately 90%[6,33]) are anteroapical, caused by infarction in the distribution of the left anterior descending coronary artery. Posterior aneurysms—aneurysms of the diaphragmatic wall occurring in the distribution of the right coronary artery—are rare, accounting for only 3%–5% of cases.[6,24] The rarity of posterior ventricular aneurysms may be due to frequent associated damage to the posterior papillary muscle and early death secondary to massive mitral regurgitation.[24]

Technique
The area of the aneurysm is not dissected until bypass is initiated and the heart is arrested. This is to diminish the possibility of dislodging an intraventricular mural thrombus.

Cardiopulmonary bypass is initiated with bicaval and ascending aortic cannulation. Single atrial cannulation with a large double-basket cannula is an alternate approach if cold cardioplegia is not used or if a limited amount of cardioplegic solution is expected to be used.

Systemic cooling is performed, the aorta is clamped, tapes are tightened around the caval cannulas, a small opening is made in the right atrium, and

Left Ventricular Aneurysm

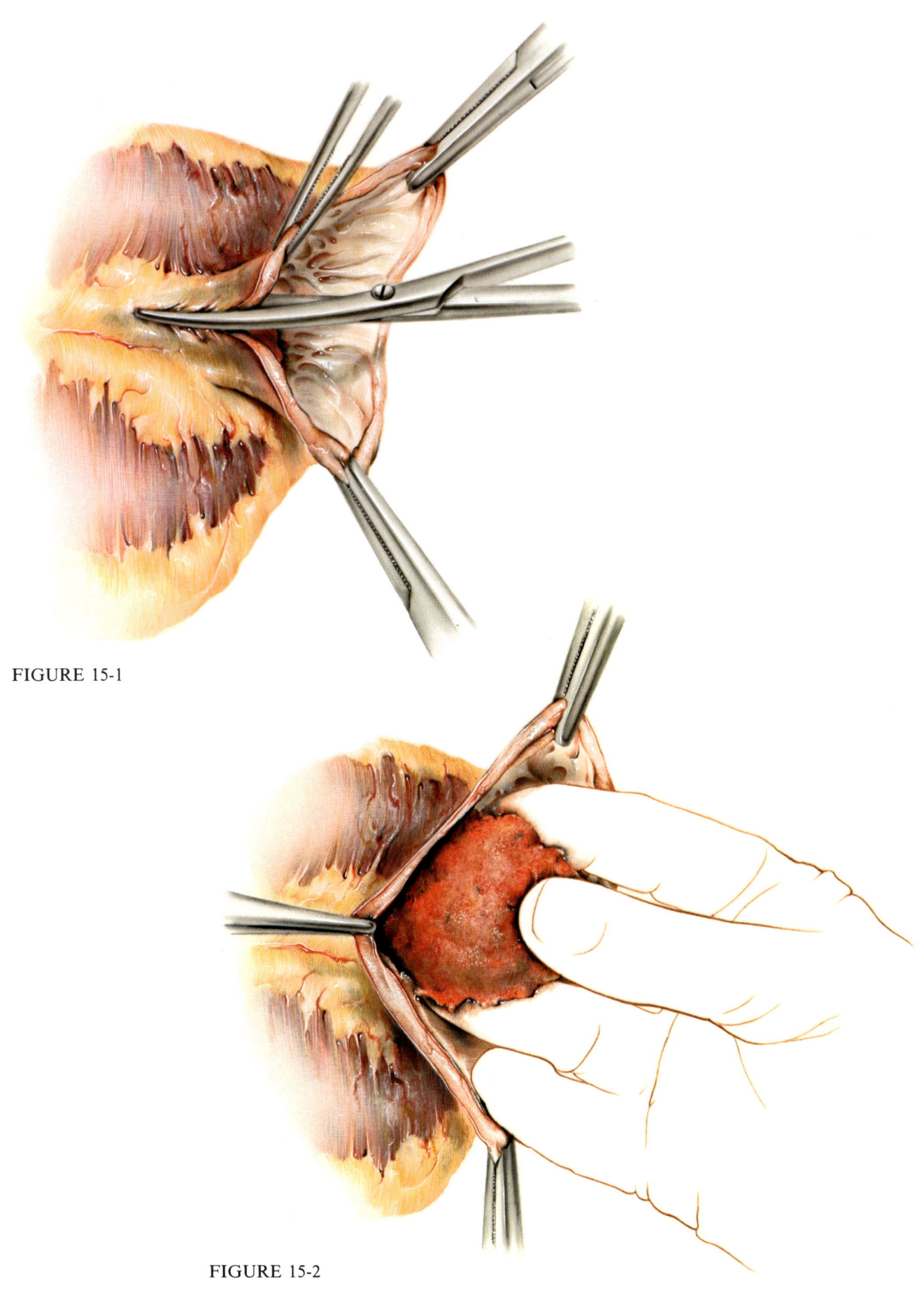

FIGURE 15-1

FIGURE 15-2

cardioplegic solution is infused into the ascending aorta. If left heart decompression is necessary, it can be accomplished through the right superior pulmonary vein or by opening the aneurysm. Myocardial temperature is measured in an area of the left ventricle that is viable, and a temperature below 15°C is sought.

The middle of the aneurysm is incised and the incision is extended with scissors (Fig. 15-1). Intramural clot is carefully scooped out (Fig. 15-2), and residual pieces are removed. Clamps placed on the edges of the aneurysm aid retraction and exposure.

At this point inspection of the interior of the left ventricle and assessment of the mitral apparatus can be done. The degree of involvement of the septum and the firmness of the septum can be determined. Although some have advocated exclusion of all infarcted septum by suturing the lateral edge of the aneurysm down to the viable septum[41,44] or buttressing of the infarcted septum with prosthetic material,[30] this has not been our general practice. Further evaluation of postoperative ventricular function and survival will be necessary to document the value of such technical modifications.[36]

Inspection of the mitral apparatus is important. Mild or moderate mitral regurgitation may be secondary to lateral "tethering" of the papillary muscles by a large aneurysm, rather than infarction of the papillary muscles or rupture of the chordae tendineae. Inspection in such an instance will show whether the disease process spares the papillary muscle and chordae. Repair of the aneurysm will usually cure the mitral regurgitation by bringing the papillary muscles back into more functional alignment.

Repair of the aneurysm is initiated by placing two wide strips of Teflon felt on each side of the aneurysm (Fig. 15-3). Horizontal mattress sutures of 0 polyester on a large (45 mm diameter) needle are taken through the felt strips and the fibrotic edges of the aneurysm. These are tied. A vent is left in the apex under the last stitch.

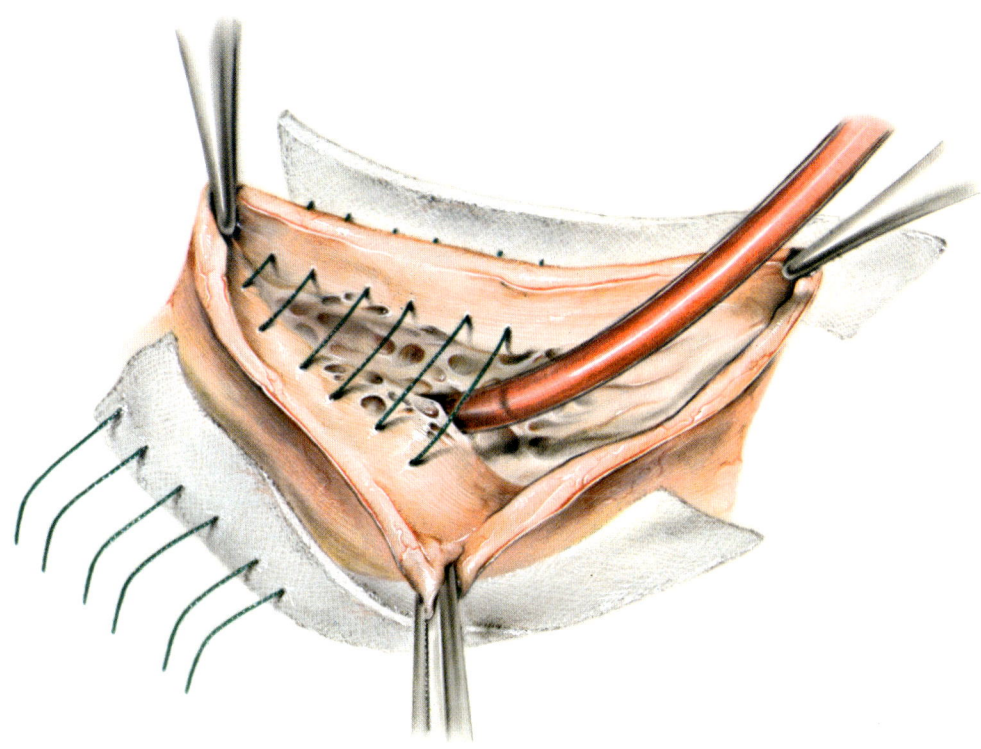

FIGURE 15-3

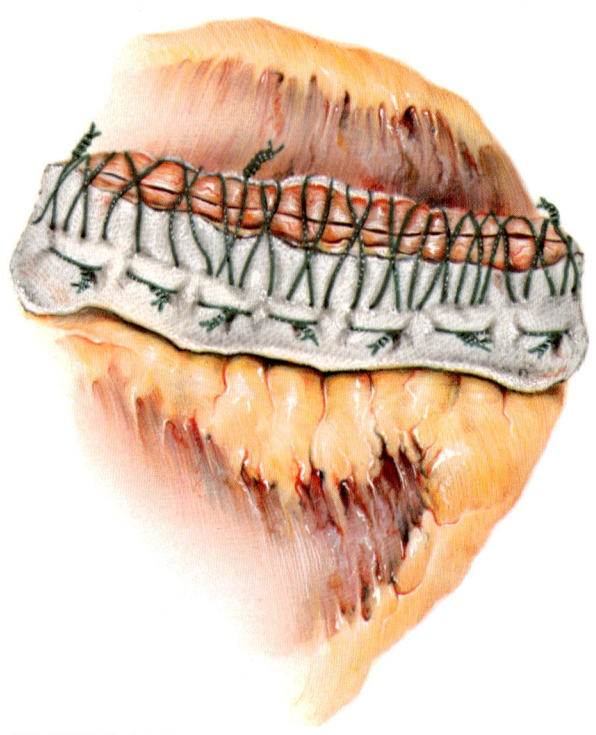

FIGURE 15-4

The edges of the aneurysm wall proturding over the Teflon strips are cut flush. A running up-and-back suture of the same 0 polyester is then taken. The aortic clamp is released as air is removed from the ascending aorta. The apex is elevated and the apical vent is partially removed to remove air and then repositioned. The heart is defibrillated if necessary, and recovery from cardioplegia is accomplished with a vented nonworking heart. The vent is then removed and several horizontal mattress sutures and simple interrupted sutures are taken at the apex to achieve complete hemostasis (Fig. 15-4). The patient is then weaned from bypass. The suture line is checked prior to removing the venous cannulas to assure hemostasis at normal systemic pressure.

Results

Operative Mortality
Operative mortality in recent reports has ranged from 3% to 11%.[6,10,19,27-29,37] This improved operative mortality is probably due to several factors: improved myocardial preservation with cold cardioplegia, better patient selection, concomitant coronary artery bypass, and resection of smaller aneurysms that are found in patients whose primary symptom is angina pectoris.

Symptomatic Improvement
The vast majority of patients undergoing surgery have improvement in symptoms, usually achieving functional class I or II status.[19] A number of reports have documented 80% or more of patients in functional class I or II.[6,27,33,37]

Ventricular Function
The results of studies of ventricular function following aneurysm resection are conflicting.[14,40] This is probably caused by different patient variables (such as extent of coronary disease), different methods of evaluating ventricular function, and different methods of selection for postoperative study. Neverthe-

less, some general statements can be made regarding changes in ventricular function following aneurysmectomy.

A majority of patients appear to have improved diastolic function postoperatively, although function does not return to normal.[40,41] Stephens and co-workers,[40] in a study of 12 patients, showed that left ventricular aneurysmectomy reduced mean left ventricular filling pressure from 25 to 17 mm Hg at rest and from 39 to 32 mm Hg during exercise, after administration of isosorbide dinitrate. Both these changes were statistically significant.

There has been little evidence that aneurysmectomy improves systolic ventricular function, at least at rest. Froehlich and colleagues,[14] studying ejection fraction by isotope ventriculogram, found an improvement by 5% or greater in only 3 of 15 patients. Stephens and colleagues,[40] measuring exercise hemodynamics by thermodilution, found no significant change in mean stroke volume index at rest or during exercise following aneurysmectomy. Functional class postoperatively appears to correlate better with ventricular filling pressure than with ventricular volume or ejection fraction.[37]

Ventricular Arrhythmia

Ventricular aneurysmectomy alone as treatment for ventricular tachyarrhythmias has had disappointing results, with persistence of arrhythmia requiring medical treatment in approximately 50% of patients.[6,10] The more rigorous the postoperative search for arrhythmias, the more arrhythmias are found. In a postoperative study of 8 patients using 24-hour ambulatory ECG, Sami and co-workers[34] found recurrent ventricular tachycardia in 5 and multifocal premature ventricular contractions in the other 3.

A new surgical technique now exists for the treatment of ventricular tachycardia: endocardial excision. Intraoperative mapping is performed to localize the area of origin of the tachycardia, which is usually at the border of the aneurysm. Endocardium is resected in the area of origin up to normal muscle. Josephson and co-workers[18] have reported results with this technique in 12 patients. Ventricular tachycardia could not be initiated by repeat electrophysiologic study postoperatively in any patient. The 10 survivors remained free of sustained ventricular tachycardia for 9–20 months, with one late nonarrhythmic death.

Survival

Most studies of the natural history of ventricular aneurysm are retrospective ones of several decades ago using autopsy data. These studies give a grim picture of the natural history of the disease. Schlicter and co-workers[35] found a three-year survival of 27% and five-year survival of 12%.

Survival data in surgically treated patients are quite good. Three-year survival calculated actuarially ranges from 71% to 81%.[29,33] Burton and colleagues[6] reported actuarial five-year survival at 60%. Surgical treatment appears to enhance survival in symptomatic patients with ventricular aneurysm.

References

1. Applebaum E, Nicholson GHB: Occlusive disease of the coronary arteries: analysis of pathological anatomy in 168 cases. Am Heart J 10:662, 1935.
2. Arthur A, Basta L, Kioschos M: Factors influencing prognosis in left ventricular aneurysmectomy. Circulation 46(Suppl II):II-127, 1972.
3. Baudet M, Rigaud M, Rocha P, Bardet J, Bourdarias JP: Treatment of early postinfarction ventricular aneurysm by intra-aortic balloon pumping and surgery. J Thorac Cardiovasc Surg 78:445, 1979.

4. Borer JS, Jacobstein JG, Bacharach SL, Green MV: Detection of left ventricular aneurysm and evaluation of effects of surgical repair: the role of radionuclide cineangiography. Am J Cardiol 45:1103, 1980.
5. Botvinick EH, Shames D, Hutchinson JC, Roe BB, Fitzpatrick M: Noninvasive diagnosis of a false left ventricular aneurysm with a radioisotope gated cardiac blood pool imaging: differentiating from true aneurysm. Am J Cardiol 37:1089, 1976.
6. Burton NA, Stinson EB, Oyer PE, Shumway NE: Left ventricular aneurysm: preoperative risk factors and long-term postoperative results. J Thorac Cardiovasc Surg 77:65, 1979.
7. Cheng TO: Incidence of ventricular aneurysm in coronary artery disease: an angiographic appraisal. Am J Med 50:340, 1971.
8. Cooley DA, Collins HA, Morris GC Jr, Chapman DW: Ventricular aneurysm after myocardial infarction: surgical excision with use of temporary cardiopulmonary bypass. JAMA 167:557, 1958.
9. Cooley DA, Norman JC: Techniques in Cardiac Surgery. Houston, Texas Medical Press, 1975, p 165.
10. Cosgrove DM, Loop FD, Irarrazaval MJ, Groves LK, Taylor PC, Golding LA: Determinants of long-term survival after ventricular aneurysmectomy. Ann Thorac Surg 26:357, 1978.
11. Dubnow MH, Burchell HB, Titus JH: Postinfarction ventricular aneurysm: a clinico-morphologic and electrocardiographic study of 80 cases. Am Heart J 70:753, 1965.
12. Dymond DS, Jarritt PH, Britton KE, Spurrell RAJ: Detection of postinfarction left ventricular aneurysms by first pass radionuclide ventriculography using a multicrystal gamma camera. Br Heart J 41:68, 1979.
13. Ersek RA, Chesler E, Korns ME, Edwards JE: Spontaneous rupture of a false left ventricular aneurysm following myocardial infarction. Am Heart J 77:677, 1969.
14. Froehlich RT, Falsetti HL, Doty DB, Marcus ML: Prospective study of surgery for left ventricular aneurysm. Am J Cardiol 45:923, 1980.
15. Gobel FL, Visudh-Arom K, Edwards JE: Pseudoaneurysm of the left ventricle leading to recurrent pericardial hemorrhage. Chest 59:23, 1971.
16. Gueron M, Wanderman KL, Hirsch M, Borman J: Pseudoaneurysm of the left ventricle after myocardial infarction: a curable form of myocardial rupture. J Thorac Cardiovasc Surg 69:736, 1975.
17. Guiraudon G, Fontaine G, Frank R, Escande G, Etievent P, Cabrol C: Encircling endocardial ventriculotomy: a new surgical treatment for life-threatening ventricular tachycardias resistant to medical treatment following myocardial infarction. Ann Thorac Surg 26:438, 1978.
18. Josephson ME, Harken AH, Horowitz LN: Endocardial excision: a new surgical technique for the treatment of recurrent ventricular tachycardia. Circulation 60:1430, 1979.
19. Kapelanski DP, Al-Sadir J, Lamberti JJ, Anagnostopoulos CE: Ventriculographic features predictive of surgical outcome for left ventricular aneurysm. Circulation 58:1167, 1978.
20. Klein MD, Herman MV, Gorlin R: A hemodynamic study of left ventricular aneurysm. Circulation 35:614, 1967.
21. Kouchoukos NT, Doty DB, Buettner LE, Kirklin JW: Treatment of postinfarction cardiac failure by myocardial excision and revascularization. Circulation 45(Suppl I):I-72, 1972.
22. Lee DC, Johnson RA, Boucher CA, Wexler LF, McEnany, MT: Angiographic predictors of survival following left ventricular aneurysmectomy. Circulation 56(Suppl II):II-12, 1977.
23. Loop FD, Effler DB, Navia JA, Sheldon WC, Groves LK: Aneurysms of the left ventricle: survival and results of a ten-year surgical experience. Ann Surg 178:399, 1973.
24. Loop FD, Effler DB, Webster JS, Groves LK: Posterior ventricular aneurysms: etiologic factors and results of surgical treatment. N Engl J Med 288:237, 1973.

25. Malcolm ID, Fitchett DH, Stewart D, Marpole D, Symes J: Ventricular aneurysm: false or true? An important distinction. Ann Thorac Surg 29:474, 1980.
26. Mirowski M, Reid PR, Mower MM, Watkins L, Gott V, Schauble JF, Langer A, Heilman MS, Kolenik SA, Fischell RE, Weisfeldt ML: Termination of malignant ventricular arrhythmias with an implanted automatic defibrillator in human beings. N Engl J Med 303:322, 1980.
27. Moran JM, Scanlon PJ, Nemickus R, Pifarre R: Surgical treatment of post-infarction ventricular aneurysm. Ann Thorac Surg 21:107, 1976.
28. Mullen DC, Posey L, Gabriel R, Singh HM, Flemma RJ, Lepley D: Prognostic considerations in the management of left ventricular aneurysms. Ann Thorac Surg 23:455, 1977.
29. Okies JE, Dietl C, Garrison HB, Starr A: Early and late results of resection of ventricular aneurysm. J Thorac Cardiovasc Surg 75:255, 1978.
30. Reul GJ: Discussion of Walker et al. J Thorac Cardiovasc Surg 76:830, 1978.
31. Rigo P, Murray M, Strauss HW, Pitt B: Scintiphotographic evaluation of patients with suspected left ventricular aneurysm. Circulation 50:985, 1974.
32. Roelandt J, Van den Brand M, Vletter WB: Echocardiographic diagnosis of pseudoaneurysm of the left ventricle. Circulation 52:466, 1975.
33. Rogers WJ, Oberman A, Kouchoukos NT: Left ventricular aneurysmectomy in patients with single vs. multivessel coronary artery disease. Circulation 58(Suppl I):I-50, 1978.
34. Sami M, Charpin D, Chabot M, Bourassa MG: Long-term follow-up of aneurysmectomy for recurrent ventricular tachycardia or fibrillation (abstr). Am J Cardiol 39:269, 1977.
35. Schlicter J, Hellerstein HK, Katz LN: Aneurysm of the heart. Correlative study of 102 proved cases. Medicine 33:43, 1954.
36. Schmidt CA, Bailey LL, Wareham EE: Septal wall motion: its significance in outcome of left ventricular scar resection. Arch Surg 115:624, 1980.
37. Shaw RC, Connors JP, Hieb BR, Ludbrook PA, Krone R, Kleigher RE, Ferguson TB, Weldon CS: Postoperative investigation of left ventricular aneurysm resection. Circulation 56(Suppl II):II-7, 1977.
38. Simpson MT, Oberman A, Kouchoukos NT, Rogers WJ: Prevalence of mural thrombi and systemic embolization with left ventricular aneurysm: effect of anticoagulation therapy. Chest 77:4, 1980.
39. Spencer FC, Green GE, Tice DA, Walsh E, Mills NL, Glassman E: Coronary artery bypass grafts for congestive heart failure: a report of experience with 40 patients. J Thorac Cardiovasc Surg 62:529, 1971.
40. Stephens JD, Dymond DS, Stone DL, Rees GM, Spurrell RAJ: Left ventricular aneurysm and congestive heart failure: value of exercise stress and isosorbide dinitrate in predicting hemodynamic results of aneurysmectomy. Am J Cardiol 45:932, 1980.
41. Stoney WS, Alford WC, Burrus GR, Thomas CS: Repair of anteroseptal ventricular aneurysm. Ann Thorac Surg 15:394, 1973.
42. Strauss HW, Zaret BL, Hurley PJ, Natarajan TK, Pitt B: A scintiphotographic method for measuring left ventricular ejection fraction in man without cardiac catheterization. Am J Cardiol 28:575, 1971.
43. Walker WE, Stoney WS, Alford WC Jr, Burrus GR, Glassford DM, Thomas CS Jr: Results of surgical management of acute left ventricular aneurysms. Circulation 62(Suppl I):I-75, 1980.
44. Walker WE, Stoney WS, Alford WC Jr, Burrus GR, Frist RA, Glassford DM, Thomas CS Jr: Techniques and results of ventricular aneurysmectomy with emphasis on anteroseptal repair. J Thorac Cardiovasc Surg 76:824, 1978.
45. Watson LE, Dickhaus DW, Martin RH: Left ventricular aneurysm: preoperative hemodynamics, chamber volume, and results of aneurysmectomy. Circulation 52:868, 1975.
46. Zaret BL, Strauss HW, Hurley PJ, Natarajan TK, Pitt B: A noninvasive scintiphotographic method for detecting regional ventricular dysfunction in man. N Engl J Med 284:1165, 1971.

16 Postinfarction Ventricular Septal Defect

Rupture of the ventricular septum is a rare but devastating complication of myocardial infarction. Recent advances in perioperative support, myocardial preservation, and technique of repair have improved surgical results in a lesion that was almost always lethal prior to the advent of surgical therapy.

Indications

Ventricular septal defect (VSD) is found in only 1%–2% of patients dying from acute myocardial infarction.[11,15] Septal rupture usually occurs from two to four days after infarction.[14,20] The natural history of the lesion is grim: approximately 25% of patients die within 24 hours, 60%–70% within two weeks, with only 10%–20% surviving two months.[18,19]

The lethal nature of postinfarction VSD stimulated the development of surgical treatment.[4] The early results indicated a lower mortality if repair was performed six or more weeks after infarction.[2] The defect rim at that stage is fibrotic and easier to repair,[16] seeming to suggest that a strategy of delay would be desirable.

However, the good results in patients operated upon weeks after infarction most likely reflect a selected group of patients with small defects and a relatively smaller amount of myocardial necrosis. The vast majority of patients die before six weeks. Therefore, delay should not be a goal. If a patient has no serious hemodynamic compromise from the development of a VSD, operation may be delayed. The vast majority of patients will require institution of circulatory support, proper study, and prompt surgery within hours or days of developing septal rupture.[5,14]

Surgical Strategy

Indications for Intraaortic Balloon Pump
Mechanical circulatory support with the intraaortic balloon pump (IABP) is a valuable advance in the management of low cardiac output secondary to septal rupture. IABP results in significant clinical and hemodynamic improvement in all cases, with a fall in the pulmonary capillary wedge pressure, a rise in mean arterial pressure, and a fall in the pulmonic/systemic flow

ratio.[3,8] Pharmacologic manipulation with nitroprusside may also help to improve hemodynamics.[22]

It is our practice to institute IABP at the first sign of depressed cardiac output and to maintain it through catheterization and the immediate postoperative period.

Myocardial Preservation

Our method of myocardial preservation is cold potassium crystalloid cardioplegia (Chapter 6).

Management of Associated Conditions

Coronary artery disease: The value of bypassing diseased coronary arteries supplying the viable myocardium has not been conclusively demonstrated.[5] Nevertheless, we feel it is likely to be beneficial and should not add any risk to the operation. For these reasons we recommend grafting any major coronary arteries that supply viable myocardium and have stenosis of 50% or more of the luminal diameter.

Mitral regurgitation: Rupture or dysfunction of the papillary muscle is associated with posterior infarction in the distribution of the right coronary artery.[6,14] Replacement of the mitral valve can be performed through the ventriculotomy.[14]

Surgical Anatomy

Approximately 70% of defects are anterior, at or near the apex.[21] Posterior defects are usually more extensive, may extend from the atrioventricular groove to the apex, and do not have as well-defined borders as anterior defects.[5,14]

Technique

Closure of Anteroapical Defect

The earliest reported repair of postinfarction VSD using cardiopulmonary bypass, by Cooley in 1957,[4] was through a right ventriculotomy. Many early repairs utilized the same approach.[1,9] The left ventricular approach, through the infarct, was increasingly advocated[7,10,12,13] and has become the preferred approach. There are several distinct advantages of the left ventricular approach over the right: (1) There are better exposure and delineation of the defect. (2) The patch is placed on the left ventricular side of the septum, with broader distribution of forces over the septum. (3) Right ventricular function is preserved.

The incision is usually made through the middle of the infarct. The loose edges of the defect are trimmed and the margins defined. A woven Dacron patch, considerably larger than the defect, is cut.

We use a modification of the double-patch technique described by Iben and colleagues.[9] This method employs broad pledgets on the right ventricular side and the patch on the left ventricular side. This is technically easier than the double-patch technique, but incorporates the same principles: broad distribution of suture force and buttressing of both sides of the septum.

Broad horizontal mattress sutures are placed with Teflon pledgets on the right ventricular side (Fig. 16-1). These are placed away from the border of the defect, in as viable muscle as is available. After all the sutures are placed, the patch is seated and tied. An additional suture line can be placed around the edge of the patch (Fig. 16-2). Closure of the ventricle is accomplished using Teflon strips, as for ventricular aneurysmectomy (Chapter 15).

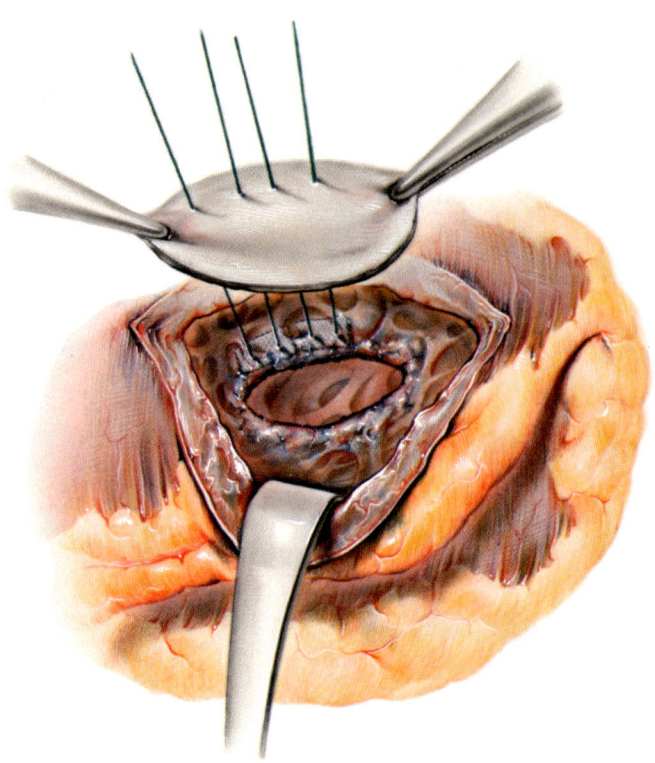

FIGURE 16-1

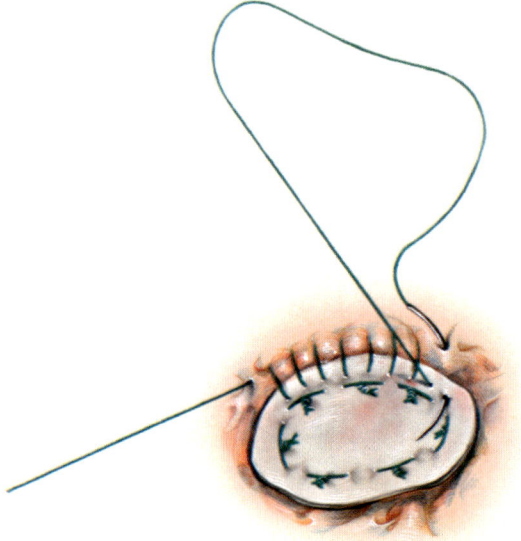

FIGURE 16-2

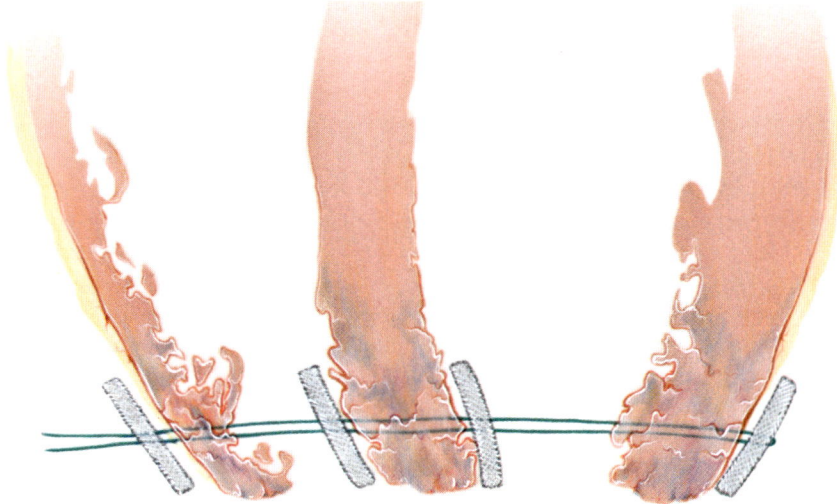

FIGURE 16-3

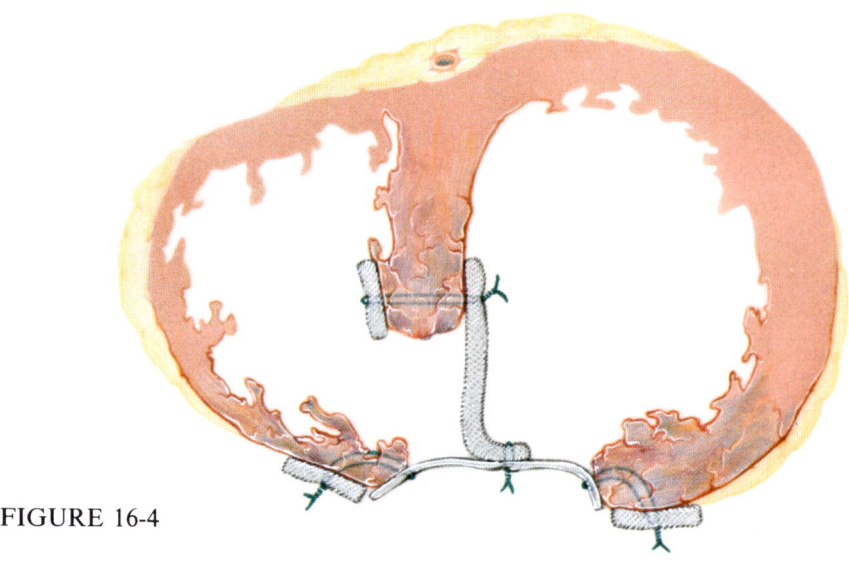

FIGURE 16-4

Alternate Methods of Repair

Modifications in repair should be made to suit the wide variety of pathologic anatomy. Repair of an anterior defect may require incorporation of part of the patch in the ventriculotomy closure. Amputation of the apex can be performed with closure of the ventricles incorporating four Teflon strips (Fig. 16-3).

Posterior defects may require extensive patching of the septum and the wall of the ventricle (Fig. 16-4), as advocated by Daggett and colleagues.[5]

Results

Operative Mortality
Overall operative mortality is in the range of 40%–50%.[5,14,17] Subgroups with higher operative mortality include those with posterior defects, those requiring valve replacement, and those in refractory cardiogenic shock.

Late Survival
The prognosis for operative survivors, at least for several years, is good. Late survival is 80%–90% two to three years postoperatively.[5,14]

References

1. Boicourt OW, Ritzmann L, Starr A, McCord CW: Rupture of the infarcted interventricular septum. Circulation 26:1321, 1962.
2. Brandt B III, Wright CB, Ehrenhaft JL: Ventricular septal defect following myocardial infarction. Ann Thorac Surg 27:580, 1979.
3. Buckley MJ, Mundth ED, Daggett WM, Gold HK, Leinbach RC, Austen WG: Surgical management of ventricular septal defect and mitral regurgitation complicating acute myocardial infarction. Ann Thorac Surg 16:598, 1973.
4. Cooley DA, Belmonte BA, Seis LB, Schnur S: Surgical repair or ruptured interventricular septum following acute myocardial infarction. Surgery 41:930, 1957.
5. Daggett WM, Guyton RA, Mundth ED, Buckley MJ, McEnany MT, Gold HK, Leinbach RC, Austen WG: Surgery for post-myocardial infarct ventricular septal defect. Ann Surg 186:260, 1977.
6. Daggett WM, Mundth ED, Gold HK, Leinbach RC, Buckley MJ, Austen WG: Early repair of ventricular septal defect complicating inferior myocardial infarction. Circulation 50(Suppl III):III-112, 1974.
7. DuBost C: Discussion of Iben AB, et al: Surgical treatment of post-infarction ventricular septal defects. Ann Thorac Surg 8:252, 1969.
8. Gold HK, Leinbach RC, Sanders CA, Buckley MJ, Mundth ED, Austen WG: Intraaortic balloon pumping for ventricular septal defect or mitral regurgitation complicating acute myocardial infarction. Circulation 47:1191, 1973.
9. Iben AB, Puppello DF, Stinson EB, Shumway NE: Surgical treatment of postinfarction ventricular septal defects. Ann Thorac Surg 8:252, 1969.
10. Javid H, Hunter JA, Najafi H, Dye WS, Julian OC: Left ventricular approach for the repair of ventricular septal perforation and infarctectomy. J Thorac Cardiovasc Surg 63:14, 1972.
11. Jonas V, Hyncik V, Chlumsky J, Chlumska A: Eight year survival after perforation of ventricular septum in myocardial infarction. Acta Univ Carol (Med) 16:133, 1970.
12. Kay JH: Discussion of Iben AB, et al: Surgical treatment of post-infarction ventricular septal defects. Ann Thorac Surg 8:252, 1969.
13. Kitamura S, Mendez A, Kay JH: Ventricular septal defect following myocardial infarction. Experience with surgical repair through a left ventriculotomy and review of literature. J Thorac Cardiovasc Surg 61:186, 1971.
14. Loisance DY, Cachera JP, Poulain H, Aubry P, Juvin AM, Galey JJ: Ventricular septal defect after acute myocardial infarction. J Thorac Cardiovasc Surg 80:61, 1980.
15. Lundberg S, Soderstrom J: Perforation of the interventricular septum in myocardial infarction: a study based upon autopsy material. Acta Med Scand 172:413, 1962.
16. Mallory GK, White PD: The speed of healing of myocardial infarction: a study of the pathologic anatomy in 72 cases. Am Heart J 18:647, 1939.
17. Naifeh JG, Grehl TM, Hurley EJ: Surgical treatment of postmyocardial infarction ventricular septal defects. J Thorac Cardiovasc Surg 79:483, 1980.
18. Oyamada A, Queen FB: Spontaneous rupture of the interventricular septum following acute myocardial infarction with some clinicopathological observations on survival in five cases. Presented at Pan Pacific Pathology Congress, Tripler US Army Hospital, 1961.
19. Sanders RJ, Kern WH, Blount SG Jr: Perforation of the interventricular septum complicating myocardial infarction: a report of eight cases, one with cardiac catheterization. Am Heart J 51:736, 1956.
20. Selzer A, Gerbode F, Kerth WJ: Clinical, hemodynamic, and surgical considerations of rupture of the ventricular septum after myocardial infarction. Am Heart J 78:598, 1969.
21. Swithinbank JM: Perforation of the interventricular septum in myocardial infarction. Br Heart J 21:562, 1959.
22. Tecklenberg PL, Fitzgerald J, Allaire BI, Alderman EL, Harrison DC: Afterload reduction in the management of postinfarction ventricular septal defect. Am J Cardiol 38:956, 1976.

Tricuspid Valve Surgery 17

The development over the past two decades of surgery for acquired disease of the tricuspid valve is characterized by steady movement away from replacement and toward techniques that conserve the valve. Replacement of the valve has become uncommon, occurring in less than 5% of patients undergoing tricuspid valve surgery. Conservative surgery of the valve—anuloplasty, occasionally in association with commissurotomy—remains an area of some controversy, involving indications for surgery, choice of anuloplasty technique, and details of technique. In this chapter we will illustrate two common methods of anuloplasty, the Carpentier and the DeVega, illustrate commissurotomy, and discuss valve replacement.

Anuloplasty

Indications

Surgery of the tricuspid valve has long been a challenge.[10,11] Methods of evaluating the severity of tricuspid insufficiency—whether clinical, hemodynamic, or operative—all involve a degree of subjectivity. The variable early results of valve repair or valve replacement led to differing recommendations regarding management of the tricuspid valve during mitral or mitral and aortic surgery, from doing nothing[3] to reparative operations[5,22] to tricuspid replacement in the majority of cases.[2,4,21,26,27] As the poor late results from tricuspid valve replacement[16] have become more apparent and the results of anuloplasty have become more predictable and reproducible, anuloplasty has become the method of choice for management of most cases of moderate to severe tricuspid insufficiency.

Tricuspid insufficiency is usually caused by right ventricular hypertension, right ventricular enlargement, and anular dilatation, secondary to mitral and/or aortic valvular disease, commonly referred to as "functional" regurgitation. It may also be caused by rheumatic disease of the anulus, valve leaflets and subvalvular mechanism—"organic" regurgitation.

The degree of regurgitation can vary from very mild, with only a soft murmur and normal right atrial pressure, to severe, with pulsating neck veins, an enlarged and pulsating liver, and right atrial hypertension. Severe regurgitation requires operative management, whereas mild regurgitation does not. The difficult decision occurs in moderate regurgitation, where clinical signs are minimal or absent, and only a slight degree of right atrial hypertension is present. Operative assessment of severity of tricuspid regurgitation is helpful in this situation.

Digital exploration of the right atrium is performed through the appendage prior to insertion of the caval cannula. The extent, width, and strength of the regurgitant jet is determined, and the valve is palpated. Operative findings can be influenced by changes in right ventricular pressure and cardiac output secondary to anesthesia and opening the chest and must be balanced with preoperative clinical and hemodynamic assessment.

Surgical Strategy

Myocardial Preservation
The usual method of myocardial preservation is cold crystalloid potassium cardioplegia (Chapter 6). This provides a still, dry field for anuloplasty. Coronary perfusion through the aortic root with the heart beating or fibrillating may also be used.

Associated Procedures
Any surgery on the mitral or aortic valve is performed prior to the tricuspid procedure.

Choice of Anuloplasty Technique
There are several anuloplasty techniques from which to choose:[30] (1) lateral anuloplasty with obliteration of the posterior leaflet, resulting in a bicuspid valve;[17,18] (2) semicircular ring anuloplasty by the method of DeVega[8] and its modifications;[1] and (3) Carpentier ring anuloplasty[5,6] and its modifications.[9,14] All techniques are capable of excellent immediate and mid-term results. It is too early to assess the superiority of one of them over the long-term. Our preference is for the DeVega or Carpentier technique.

Surgical Anatomy
The three leaflets of the tricuspid valve are the anterior, posterior, and septal (Fig. 17-1). There are two main papillary muscles supporting the valve: the *anterolateral,* with chordae tendineae inserting on the anterior and posterior leaflets, and the *posteromedial,* with chordae inserting on the septal leaflet.

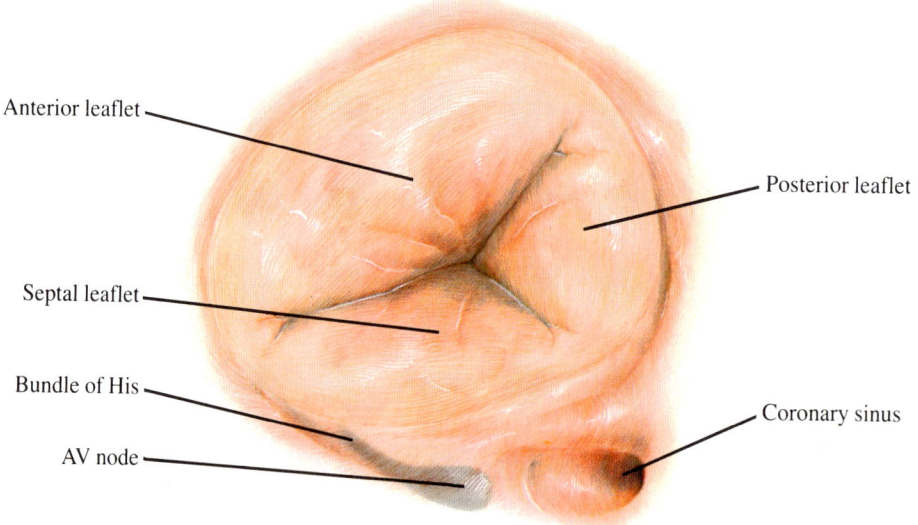

FIGURE 17-1

The atrioventricular (AV) node is located just medial to the orifice of the coronary sinus. The bundle of His begins as a continuation of the AV node at the right fibrous trigone, also called the central fibrous body: the confluence of the AV valves, atrial septum, membranous ventricular septum, and aortic valve ring. The His bundle pierces the membranous ventricular septum or skirts the septum posteriorly to enter the summit of the muscular ventricular septum, where it gives off multiple branches to the left ventricle.[15,29]

Technique

DeVega Anuloplasty

A suture of 2-0 polypropylene is passed through a pledget of Teflon, and the suture line is begun near the commissure between the anterior and septal leaflets (Fig. 17-2). Bites are taken just into or near the anulus as the suture line proceeds laterally around the anterior leaflet.

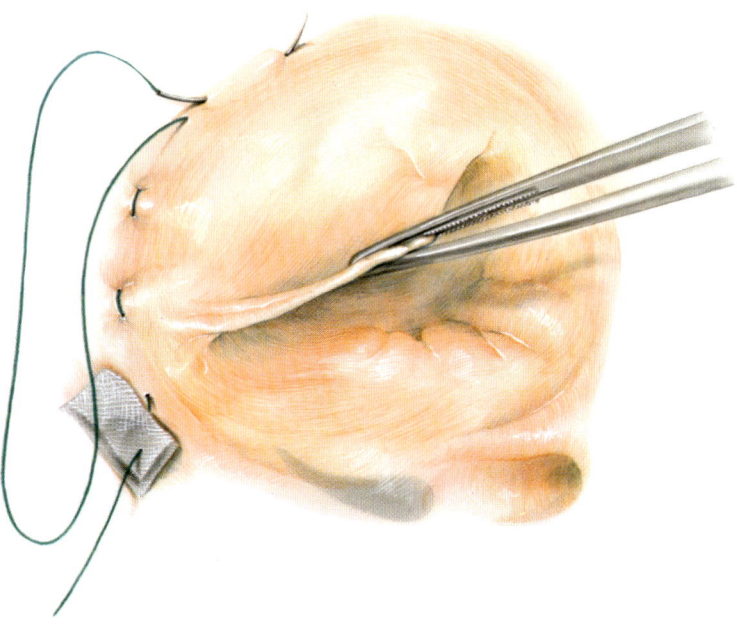

FIGURE 17-2

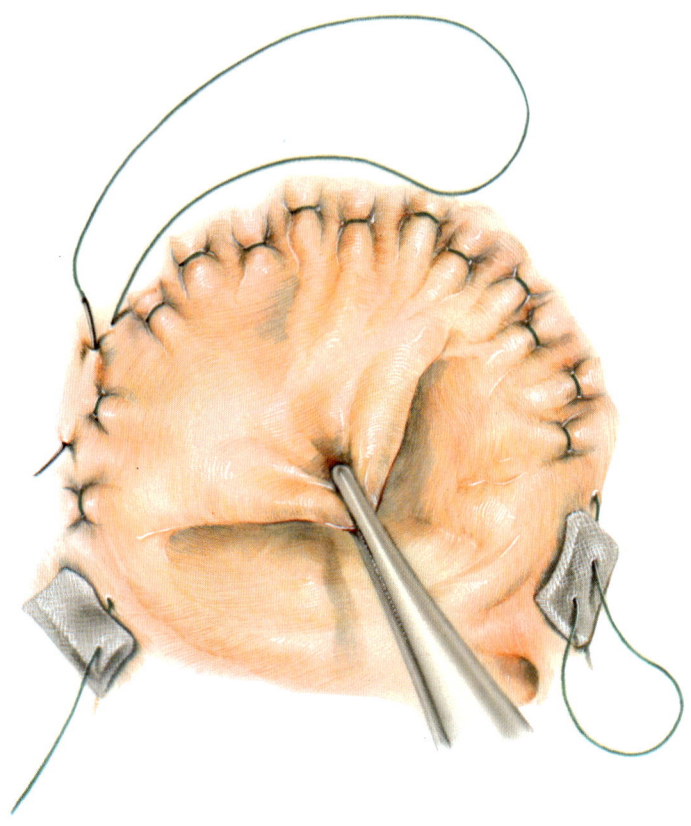

FIGURE 17-3

Near the commissure between the posterior and septal leaflets the suture is passed through another Teflon pledget and is carried back to its origin, taking bites just outside the inner suture line (Fig. 17-3).

A valve sizer appropriate to the patient's size is placed in the anulus for calibration. The suture is then tied over the medial pledget as the suture is gathered and anulus is brought against the sizer. The competence of the valve is assessed by injecting cold saline into the right ventricle with a large bulb syringe.

Carpentier Ring Anuloplasty

Coauthored by Alain Carpentier

The basis of the Carpentier ring anuloplasty is anulus remodeling: both dilatation and deformation are corrected. Right ventricular volume and pressure overload cause a change in shape of the tricuspid anulus as well as in size: the anulus becomes circular, losing its normal ovoid shape.[6,7,13] This change in shape moves the anterior and posterior leaflets out of apposition with each other and with the septal leaflet. Implantation of the Carpentier ring brings the anular shape back toward normal. The aim is to correct the tricuspid insufficiency by creating a valve orifice with normal morphology without any appreciable narrowing of the orifice.

Use of the ring allows plication of the anulus where the dilatation is most prominent—at the commissures. The ring is flexible, with a large opening at the anteroseptal commissure and septal leaflet, preventing injury to the bundle of His.

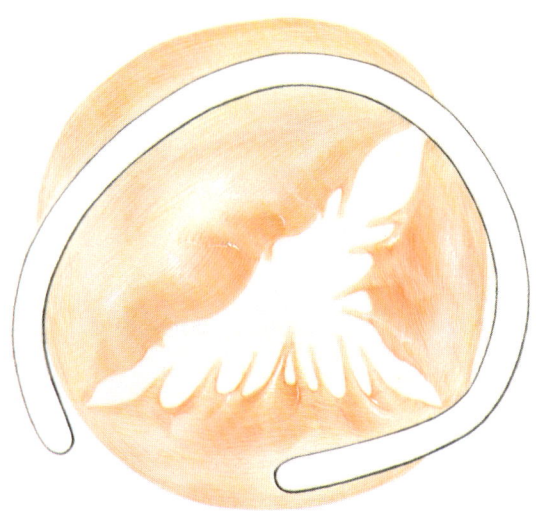

FIGURE 17-4

The size of the ring is chosen either by measurement at the base of the septal leaflet, which is not affected by anular dilatation, or by fitting the ring to the size of the anterior leaflet (Fig. 17-4). Horizontal mattress sutures are then placed in the anulus and through the fabric of the ring (Fig. 17-5). Plication takes place at the commissures. The ring is seated and tied (Fig. 17-6). Competence of the valve is checked by injecting saline into the right ventricle with a large bulb syringe.

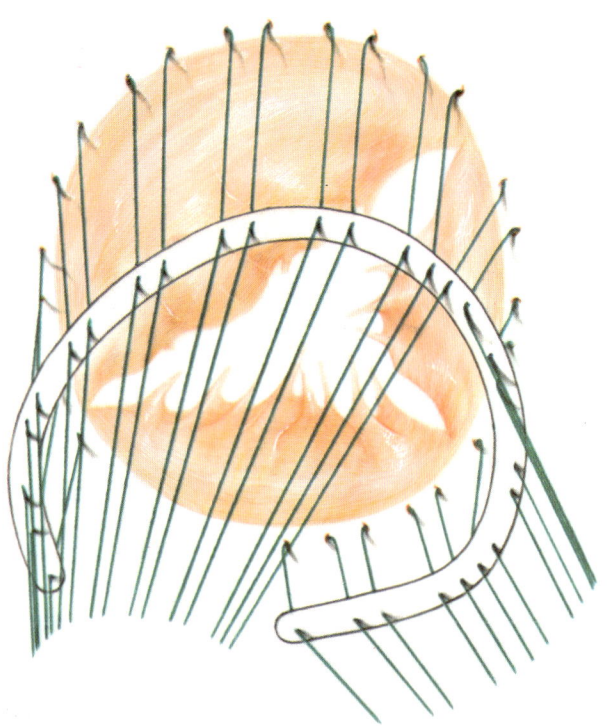

FIGURE 17-5

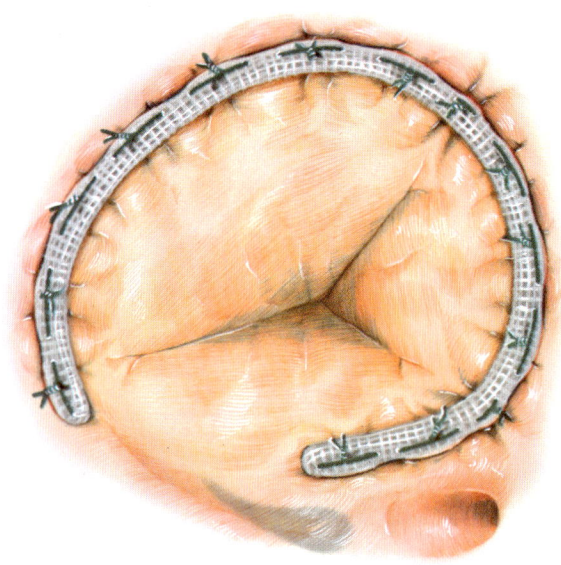

FIGURE 17-6

Results

Contemporary operative mortality is in the range of 5%–15%.[8,18] Good functional and hemodynamic results have been reported with a number of techniques.[5,8,9,11,14,17,18] Grondin and colleagues[11] reported 17 patients studied after a DeVega anuloplasty and 32 studied after Carpentier ring anuloplasty. Tricuspid insufficiency was absent or trivial in 75%, even in the presence of elevated right ventricular pressures. The DeVega technique may be less predictable than the ring technique and can create tricuspid stenosis.[12,20]

Commissurotomy

Indications

Organic tricuspid valve disease is becoming rare in the United States and many European countries. In other areas of the world, however, it is quite common.

Organic involvement of the valve can create stenosis by fusion of the commissures. Stenosis is usually part of a mixed lesion including regurgitation. Most valves with stenosis can be repaired with commissurotomy and anuloplasty. Any valve with more than a 5 mm Hg gradient should be explored.

Technique

The commissures are incised with a knife to within about 3 mm of the anulus (Fig. 17-7). Usually nothing needs to be done to the chordae. An anuloplasty should be performed to correct the insufficiency. The use of a prosthetic ring in this situation is important to avoid narrowing of the orifice.

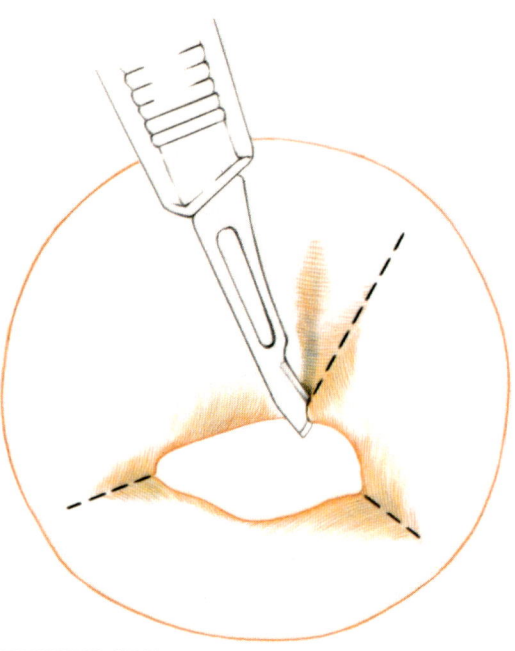

FIGURE 17-7

Replacement

Indications

Traumatic injury of the tricuspid valve is usually an indication for replacement.[28] In rare instances, leaflet tears may be repaired. Symptoms may not occur until many years following injury. Tricuspid valve replacement is also indicated in most symptomatic patients with Ebstein's disease.[19] Replacement may be indicated in symptomatic patients late after tricuspid valve excision for endocarditis.

Replacement for organic or functional tricuspid disease is rarely indicated. A less than perfect repair is preferable to replacement. An insufficient valve should be replaced only if there is rupture of multiple chordae or other irreparable damage. A valve with mixed stenosis and insufficiency should be replaced only if the chronic inflammation and scarring are so extensive that the leaflets are shrunken and curled and the chordae are thickened and shortened.

Surgical Strategy

Choice of Prosthesis

Mechanical prostheses in the tricuspid position are prone to thrombotic obstruction.[16,23,24] The struts of caged-ball valves frequently penetrate the right ventricular endocardium, resulting in restriction of ball excursion. This is usually a gradual process. Tilting-disc valves may have restriction of disc movement due to thrombus formation; this can cause catastrophic malfunction. The wedge-shaped right ventricular cavity conforms poorly to both types of mechanical prosthesis.

Our preference is for a bioprosthesis. The bioprostheses, with central flow and absence of areas prone to thrombus formation and propagation, are likely to provide superior performance in the tricuspid position, at least over the short term (three to eight years).

Technique

The valve is excised, leaving about 4 mm of the base of the septal leaflet. Horizontal mattress sutures with pledgets on the atrial side are placed in the anulus of the anterior and posterior leaflets. The sutures are placed through leaflet tissue of the septal leaflet, in order to avoid injury to the His bundle. Heart block can be an early or late complication, and we leave permanent epicardial leads whenever tricuspid valve replacement is performed.

Results

Replacement of the tricuspid valve, in association with replacement of the mitral and/or aortic valves, can be performed with operative mortality as low as 10%–15%.[4,27] Functional improvement occurs in 85%–95%.[16,23] Late survival is variable, but can be as high as 70% at three years.[23]

References

1. Alonso-Lej F: Discussion of Duran et al: Clinical and hemodynamic performance of a totally flexible prosthetic ring for atrioventricular valve reconstruction. Ann Thorac Surg 22:463, 1976.
2. Boyd AD, Engelman RM, Isom OW, Reed GE, Spencer FC: Tricuspid annuloplasty: five and one-half years' experience with 78 patients. J Thorac Cardiovasc Surg 68:344, 1974.
3. Braunwald NS, Ross J Jr, Morrow AG: Conservative management of tricuspid regurgitation in patients undergoing mitral valve replacement. Circulation 35(Suppl I):I-63, 1967.

4. Breyer RH, McClenathan JH, Michaelis LL, McIntosh CL, Morrow AG: Tricuspid regurgitation: a comparison of nonoperative management, tricuspid annuloplasty, and tricuspid valve replacement. J Thorac Cardiovasc Surg 72:867, 1976.
5. Carpentier A, Deloche A, Hanania G, Forman J, Sellier P, Piwnica A, Dubost C: Surgical management of acquired tricuspid valve disease. J Thorac Cardiovasc Surg 67:53, 1974.
6. Carpentier A, Relland J: Carpentier rings and tricuspid insufficiency (letter). Ann Thorac Surg 27:95, 1979.
7. Deloche A, Guerinon J, Fariani JM, Morillo F, Caramanian M, Carpentier A, Maurice P, Dubost C: Etude anatomique des valvuloplasties rhumatismales tricuspidiennes. Arch Mal Coeur 67:5, 1974.
8. DeVega NG: La anuloplastia selectiva, reguable y permanente. Rev Esp Cardiol 25:6, 1972.
9. Duran CG, Ubago JLM: Clinical and hemodynamic performance of a totally flexible prosthetic ring for atrioventricular valve reconstruction. Ann Thorac Surg 22:458, 1976.
10. Grondin P, Lepage G, Castongnay Y, Meere C: The tricuspid valve: a surgical challenge. J Thorac Cardiovasc Surg 53:7, 1967.
11. Grondin P, Meere C, Limet R, Lopez-Bescos L, Delcan JL, Rivera R: Carpentier's annulus and DeVega's annuloplasty: the end of the tricuspid challenge. J Thorac Cardiovasc Surg 70:852, 1975.
12. Haerten K, Seipel L, Loogen F, Herzer J: Hemodynamic studies after DeVega's tricuspid anuloplasty. Circulation 58(Suppl I):I-28, 1978.
13. Hansing CE, Rowe GG: Tricuspid insufficiency. A study of hemodynamics and pathogenesis. Circulation 45:793, 1972.
14. Hecart J, Blaise C, Bex JP, Bajolet A: Technique for tricuspid annuloplasty with a flexible linear reducer. J Thorac Cardiovasc Surg 79:689, 1980.
15. James TN: Morphology of the human atrioventricular node, with remarks pertinent to its electrophysiology. Am Heart J 62:756, 1961.
16. Jugdutt BI, Fraser RS, Lee SJK, Rossall RE, Callaghan JC: Long-term survival after tricuspid valve replacement. J Thorac Cardiovasc Surg 74:20, 1977.
17. Kay JH, Masselli-Campagna G, Tusju HK: Surgical treatment of tricuspid insufficiency. Ann Surg 162:53, 1965.
18. Kay JH, Mendez AM, Zubiate P: A further look at tricuspid annuloplasty. Ann Thorac Surg 22:498, 1976.
19. Melo J, Saylam A, Knight R, Starr A: Long-term results after surgical correction of Ebstein's anomaly. J Thorac Cardiovasc Surg 78:233, 1979.
20. Meyer J, Bircks W: Predictable correction of tricuspid insufficiency by semicircular annuloplasty. Ann Thorac Surg 23:574, 1977.
21. Pluth JR, Ellis FH Jr: Tricuspid insufficiency in patients undergoing mitral valve replacement: conservative management, annuloplasty, or replacement. J Thorac Cardiovasc Surg 58:484, 1969.
22. Reed GE, Boyd AD, Spencer FC, Engelman RM, Isom OW, Cunningham JN: Operative management of tricuspid regurgitation. Circulation 54(Suppl III):III-96, 1976.
23. Sanfelippo PM, Giuliani ER, Danielson GK, Wallace RB, Pluth JR, McGoon DC: Tricuspid valve prosthetic replacement: early and late results with the Starr-Edwards prosthesis. J Thorac Cardiovasc Surg 71:441, 1976.
24. Schoevaerdts JC, Jaumin P, Piret L, Kremer R, Ponlot R, Chalant CH: Tricuspid valve surgery. J Cardiovasc Surg 18:397, 1977.
25. Silver MD, Lam JHC, Ranganathan N, Wigle ED: Morphology of the human tricuspid valve. Circulation 43:333, 1971.
26. Starr A: Acquired disease of the tricuspid valve. In Sabiston DC Jr, Spencer FC (eds): Gibbon's Surgery of the Chest. Philadelphia, WB Saunders Co, 1976, p 1176.
27. Starr A, Herr RH, Wood JA: Tricuspid replacement for acquired valve disease. Surg Gynecol Obstet 122:1295, 1966.

28. Tachovsky TJ, Giuliani ER, Ellis FH Jr: Prosthetic valve replacement for traumatic tricuspid insufficiency. Am J Cardiol 26:196, 1970.
29. Titus JL: Normal anatomy of the human cardiac conductive system. Mayo Clin Proc 48:23, 1973.
30. West PN, Weldon CS: Reconstructive valve surgery. Ann Thorac Surg 25:167, 1978.

18 Pulmonary Valve Stenosis

This chapter deals with obstruction at the level of the pulmonary valve with an intact ventricular septum. The obstruction may be caused by valvular stenosis or atresia and is often accompanied by a variable degree of infundibular muscular stenosis. Pulmonary stenosis or atresia presenting in the neonatal period can be a difficult problem. Moderate to severe pulmonary stenosis presenting in the child or adult can usually be managed by a simple, low-risk operation.

Pulmonary Valvotomy

Indications for Surgery and Choice of Operation

Neonate
Pulmonary stenosis or atresia presenting in the first days of life is uncommon, but is lethal without surgical treatment. Pulmonary blood flow is dependent upon the ductus; and as the ductus closes, these patients present with severe cyanosis and acidosis. The difficulty in management of this condition is reflected in the number and variety of surgical approaches.[1,6,9,13,19,21] Increasing knowledge of the anatomic subsets of pulmonary stenosis or atresia and the recent use of prostaglandin E_1 have made management of this condition simpler and more predictable.

The anatomy and size of the right ventricle are critical in determining surgical management. Greenwold[5,11] has classified these ventricles into two types: I and II. Type I has a diminutive right ventricular cavity and frequently has myocardial sinusoids, which on right ventriculogram may fill the coronary arteries with retrograde opacification of the aorta.[14] Type II has a normal-sized right ventricle. Dobbell and Grignon[6] have suggested further division of type I into IA (threadlike or no passageway through the conus) and IB (ventricular cavity extending up to the atretic valve).

Our management[10] of pulmonary stenosis or atresia in type IB or type II ventricles is valvotomy without shunt, preferably under direct vision and cardiopulmonary bypass, with perioperative maintenance of ductal patency with prostaglandin E_1. A patch across the right ventricular outflow tract is avoided. Valvectomy is performed only in rare instances.[7,22] Closed valvotomy can also give excellent results.[6] Type IA may require a systemic-pulmonary shunt, either a Waterston or a polytetrafluoroethylene tube.

It is not necessary nor is it always possible to drop right ventricular pressure to below systemic levels or to raise arterial oxygen levels to normal. What can be predictably accomplished is an increase of pulmonary blood flow to levels that allow arterial oxygen tension consistent with survival. After valvotomy the oxygen tension gradually rises as right ventricular compliance increases, right ventricular volume increases, and right ventricular filling pressure drops—all resulting in a reduction in the right-to-left shunt at the atrial level.

Valvotomy in the neonatal period seldom results in permanent relief of stenosis. Repeat valvotomy, frequently with patch enlargement of the pulmonary anulus (a low-risk procedure at that time), is usually necessary within the first three years of life.[9] Of note, late tricuspid disease has not occurred when valvotomy is performed as the initial operation.

Child and Adult

Pulmonary stenosis can cause easy fatigability, dyspnea on exertion, or cyanosis on exertion or at rest. It also may be asymptomatic.[4] We consider a gradient of 80 mm Hg or more or right ventricular pressure over 100 mm Hg to be an indication for surgery. Gradients between 50 and 80 must be considered on an individual basis. Gradients less than 50 mm Hg can be tolerated well for years and are not usually an indication for surgery.[12]

Surgical Strategy

Myocardial Preservation

Coronary perfusion through the aortic root with electrically induced ventricular fibrillation is the usual method.

Management of the Foramen Ovale

A patulous foramen ovale is seldom closed. However, a significant atrial defect should be excluded, either preoperatively by echocardiography or at the time of operation by palpation or inspection. The foramen ovale is never closed in neonates, since closure would prevent decompression of the right side of the heart.

Transanular Patch

The method of determining the necessity of a transanular patch during tetralogy of Fallot repair (Chapter 22), as described by Pacifico, Kirklin, and Blackstone,[16] is also applicable to isolated pulmonary stenosis. This method bases the decision for enlargement of the pulmonary valve ring on a weight-related or surface area-related "minimum pulmonary valve ring diameter." This method is based on the studies of normal pulmonary anulus size by Rowlatt, Rimoldi, and Lev.[18]

Calibrated dilators are passed through the pulmonary valve from above. If valvotomy does not result in a normal or near-normal pulmonary diameter, the incision is extended across the anulus and a patch is placed. The chart of Pacifico and colleagues is also useful for determining the size of the patch. We do not usually place transanular patches in neonates, expecting that they will need a second operation.

Infundibular Resection

Marked infundibular hypertrophy occurs in approximately 50% of cases of pulmonary stenosis. However, infundibular resection or patching is rarely needed. The infundibular stenosis is usually dynamic and resolves after relief of the valvular stenosis.

The ventriculogram should be carefully assessed to determine the state of the infundibulum throughout the cardiac cycle. The dynamic basis of the infundibular stenosis is demonstrated by relaxation and wide opening of the infundibular region during diastole.

At operation the infundibulum is exposed through the valve after valvotomy. Inspection usually reveals no evidence of infundibular fibrosis or fixed narrowing. The probes that are passed through the valve are also passed through the infundibulum into the right ventricle. They should pass with little, if any, resistance. If fibrosis or fixed resistance is found, infundibular muscle is resected through the pulmonary valve or, more likely, by ventriculotomy with patch graft. We have found resection to be necessary in less than 10% of cases.

Surgical Technique

Closed Valvotomy

Closed valvotomy was the original surgical approach for pulmonary stenosis,[2,3,20] The instruments that we use for closed valvotomy are shown in Figure 18-1. These include a sharp instrument to perforate the valve and clamps which are spread to tear open the valve.

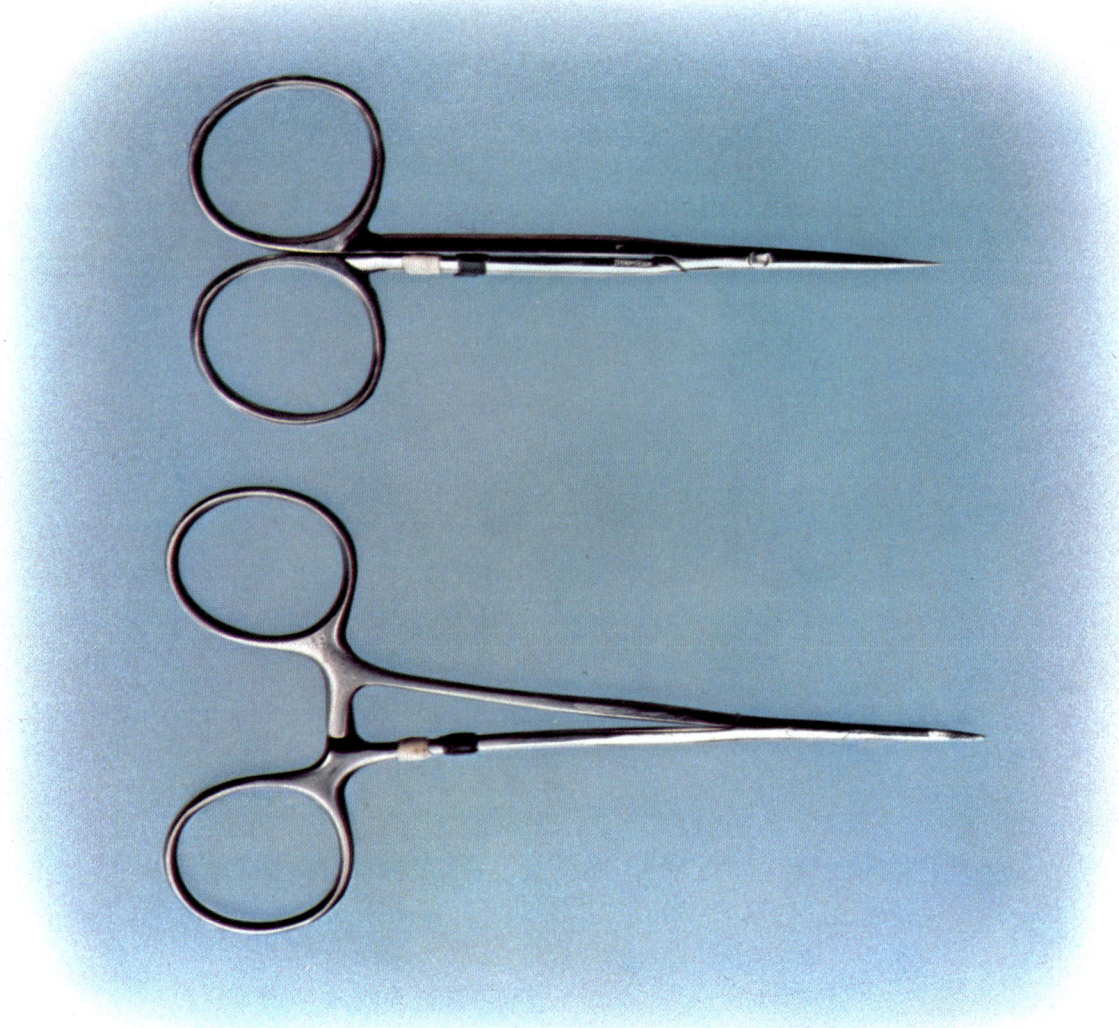

FIGURE 18-1

A purse-string suture of polypropylene is placed in the infundibulum. The sharp instrument is used to perforate the valve if the valve is atretic. The spreading instrument is then placed in the valve. Proper position can be confirmed by palpation through the pulmonary artery. The instrument is then opened. A "pop" or tearing of the valve can usually be felt. Closed valvotomy should create an easily palpable thrill over the pulmonary artery.

Open Valvotomy
Total cardiopulmonary bypass is instituted, the heart is electically fibrillated, and a cardiotomy sucker is placed in the right atrium for coronary sinus return. Retraction sutures are placed in the infundibulum just below the valve, and the main pulmonary artery is opened longitudinally. Leaflet retractors are placed exposing the valve, which is usually tricuspid with fusion of all three commissures. The commissures are incised sharply back to the anulus (Figs. 18-2, 18-3). The infundibulum is then inspected, and the valve diameter and infundibulum are calibrated as previously discussed.

Results

Neonate
Operative mortality as high as 75% has been reported for pulmonary atresia or stenosis in the neonate.[23] However, operative mortality as low as 9%–14% can be achieved in types IB and II.[6,9] Late survival is good, with actuarial survival at our institution of 77% at one year and seven years. Growth of the right ventricle can be dramatic, with as much as doubling in size.[8,15,17] As noted earlier, a second operation during the first three years of life is frequently necessary.[9]

Child and Adult
The operative risk of open valvotomy in acyanotic patients is less than 1%. Symptom relief and late survival are excellent.[4]

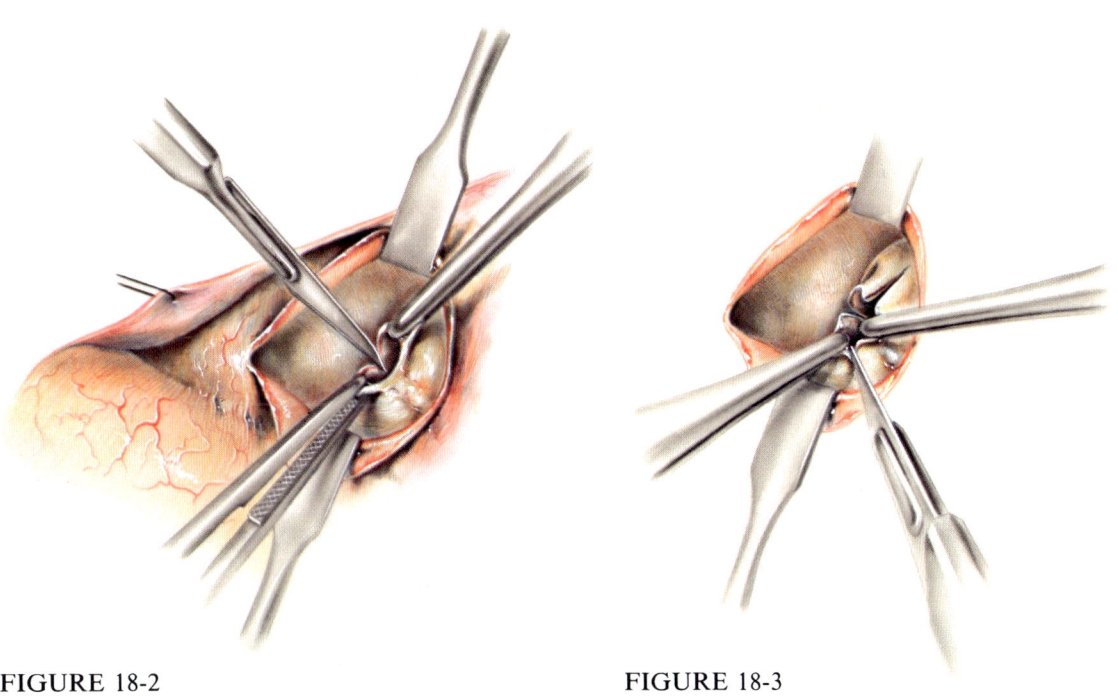

FIGURE 18-2   FIGURE 18-3

References

1. Bowman FO, Malm JR, Hayes CJ, Gersony WM, Ellis K: Pulmonary atresia with intact ventricular septum. J Thorac Cardiovasc Surg 61:85, 1971.
2. Brock RC: Pulmonary valvulotomy for the relief of congenital pulmonary stenosis: report of three cases. Br Med J 1:1121, 1948.
3. Brock RC Campbell M: Valvulotomy for pulmonary valvular stenosis. Br Heart J 12:377, 1950.
4. Danielson GK, Exarhos ND, Weidman WH, McGoon DC: Pulmonic stenosis with intact ventricular septum. J Thorac Cardiovasc Surg 61:228, 1971.
5. Davingnon AL, Greenwold WE, DuShane JW, Edwards JE: Congenital pulmonary atresia with intact ventricular septum: clinicopathological correlation of two anatomic types. Am Heart J 62:591, 1961.
6. Dobell ARC, Grignon A: Early and late results in pulmonary atresia. Ann Thorac Surg 24:264, 1977.
7. Edmunds LH Jr: Pulmonary valvular dysplasia (editorial). Ann Thorac Surg 24:498, 1977.
8. Freed MD, Rosenthal A, Bernhard WF, Litwin SB, Nadas AS: Critical pulmonary stenosis with a diminutive right ventricle in neonates. Circulation 48:875, 1973.
9. Gomez-Engler HE, Grunkemeier GL, Starr A: Critical pulmonary valve stenosis with intact ventricular septum. Thorac Cardiovasc Surg 27:160, 1979.
10. Gomez-Engler HE, Nichols GM, Sunderland C, Kirby W, Lees MH, Starr A: The role of prostaglandin E_1 and valvotomy in the treatment of critical pulmonary valve obstruction with intact ventricular septum (abstr). Circulation 60(Suppl II):II-169, 1979.
11. Greenwold WE: A clinico-pathological study of congenital tricuspid atresia and pulmonary stenosis or atresia with intact ventricular septum. Thesis, Graduate School, University of Minnesota, 1955.
12. Johnson LW, Grossman W, Dalen JE, Dexter L: Pulmonic stenosis in the adult: long-term follow-up results. N Engl J Med 287:1159, 1972.
13. Luckstead EF, Mattioli L, Reed WA, Diehl AM: Two-stage palliative surgical approach for pulmonary atresia with intact ventricular septum (type I). Am J Cardiol 29:490, 1972.
14. Miller GAH, Restifo M, Shinebourne EA, Paneth M, Joseph MC, Lennox SC, Kerr IH: Pulmonary atresia with intact ventricular septum and critical pulmonary stenosis presenting in first month of life. Br Heart J 35:9, 1973.
15. Moller JH, Girod D, Amplatz K, Varco RL: Pulmonary valvotomy in pulmonary atresia with hypoplastic right ventricle. Surgery 68:730, 1970.
16. Pacifico AD, Kirklin JW, Blackstone EH: Surgical management of pulmonary stenosis in tetralogy of Fallot. J Thorac Cardiovasc Surg 74:382, 1977.
17. Rao PS, Liebman J, Borkat G: Right ventricular growth in a case of pulmonic stenosis with intact ventricular septum and hypoplastic right ventricle. Circulation 53:389, 1976.
18. Rowlatt UF, Rimoldi HJA, Lev M: The quantitative anatomy of the normal child's heart. Pediatr Clin North Am 10:499, 1963.
19. Rudolph AM, Heyman MA, Fishman N, Lakier JB: Formalin infiltration of the ductus arteriosus: a method for palliation of infants with selected congenital cardiac lesions. N Engl J Med 292:1263, 1975.
20. Sellors TH: Surgery of pulmonary stenosis: a case in which the pulmonary valve was successfully divided. Lancet 1:988, 1948.
21. Trusler GA, Fowler RS: The surgical management of pulmonary atresia with intact ventricular septum and hypoplastic right ventricle. J Thorac Cardiovasc Surg 59:740, 1970.
22. Watkins L, Donahoo JS, Harrington D, Haller JA, Neill CA: Surgical management of congenital pulmonary valve dysplasia. Ann Thorac Surg 24:498, 1977.
23. Willis WH: Discussion of Dobell et al: Early and late results in pulmonary atresia. Ann Thorac Surg 24:264, 1977.

Atrial Septal Defects 19

Atrial septal defect (ASD) was the first cardiac malformation to be successfully treated surgically using the mechanical pump oxygenator. Following Gibbon's pioneering report,[11] surgical risk for closure of most defects became minimal and has been near 0% for the past two decades. Indications for surgery and surgical techniques for the three main types of defects—sinus venosus, ostium secundum, and ostium primum—are straightforward and widely accepted.

Indications for Surgery

Ostium secundum defects account for approximately 70% of ASDs, ostium primum defects for approximately 20%, and sinus venosus defects for approximately 10%.[25] Ostium primum defects usually cause symptoms in childhood,[22] but all types usually become symptomatic by the fourth decade of life,[5,19] usually associated with massive right ventricular dilatation, right ventricular failure, and chronic atrial fibrillation. Premature death during the fourth and fifth decades is common.[3-5,9,23]

The extremely low risk of surgical closure and excellent results justify closure if a left-to-right shunt of 1.5:1 or more is present. Closure should be performed during the first decade, preferably before school age, even in the absence of symptoms. Rarely, an isolated secundum ASD will require closure in infancy.[18]

ASD is the most common congenital cardiac lesion presenting in adulthood. The vast majority of adults with ASDs should have closure and good results should be achieved.[12] However, pulmonary hypertension (pulmonary artery systolic pressure over 60 mm Hg) may have developed and may affect the decision regarding surgery. In the presence of pulmonary hypertension, a shunt of at least 1.5:1 should be present for closure.[1] Closure should probably not be performed if the pulmonary vascular resistance is over 8 units. A continuous right-to-left shunt is an absolute contraindication to closure.

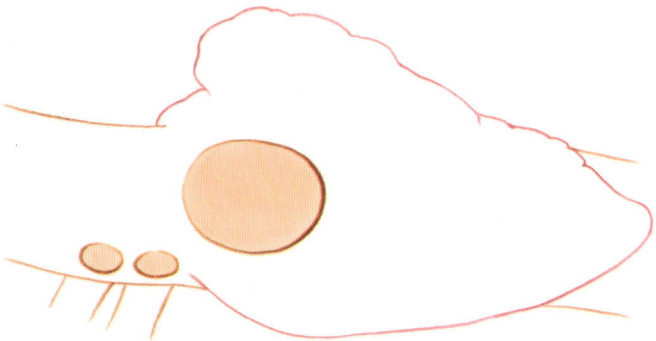

FIGURE 19-1

Sinus Venosus Defect

Surgical Anatomy
The sinus venosus defect[20] is in the upper artrial septum, above the fossa ovalis and separate from it[8] (Fig. 19-1). Anomalous pulmonary veins from the right upper lobe are almost always present and usually empty into the superior vena cava (SVC).

Surgical Technique
Our technique is similar to that described by Kirklin, Ellis, and Wood.[14] Proper surgical technique will result in complete closure while avoiding the complications of sinus node injury, pulmonary vein obstruction, and obstruction of the SVC.[24]

The SVC is carefully dissected to well above the pericardium prior to cannulation, identifying the site of entry of the anomalous pulmonary veins and the azygos vein. The azygos vein is encircled and tied. The SVC is encircled with a tape above the azygos vein. Placement of the tape above the azygos vein avoids injury to the sinus node and provides adequate exposure of the upper margin of the defect and the orifices of the pulmonary veins. Cannulation is performed using a small cannula in the SVC. The method of myocardial preservation is coronary perfusion through the aortic root at normothermia with electrically induced ventricular fibrillation.

The right atriotomy is made and extended laterally up the SVC; lateral incision is important to avoid injury to the sinus node (Fig. 19-2). The SVC cannula is retracted anteriorly.

A patch of Dacron is then cut to provide a baffle for closure of the defect and direction of pulmonary venous blood into the left atrium via the ASD. The ASD may need enlarging in some cases. A running suture of 4-0 or 5-0 polypropylene is started medially and carried along the upper portion of the defect and laterally (Fig. 19-3). Large bites medially can injure the sinus node or sinus node artery.

The inferior suture line is then brought laterally to complete the repair (Fig. 19-4). If there is any question about SVC obstruction by the baffle, the SVC should be patched with pericardium,[21] although this is seldom necessary.

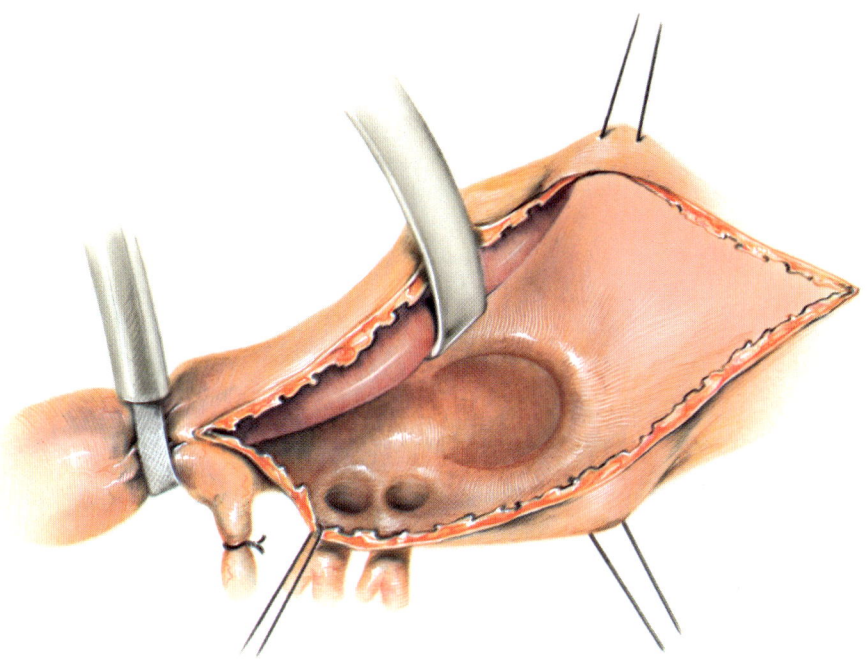

FIGURE 19-2

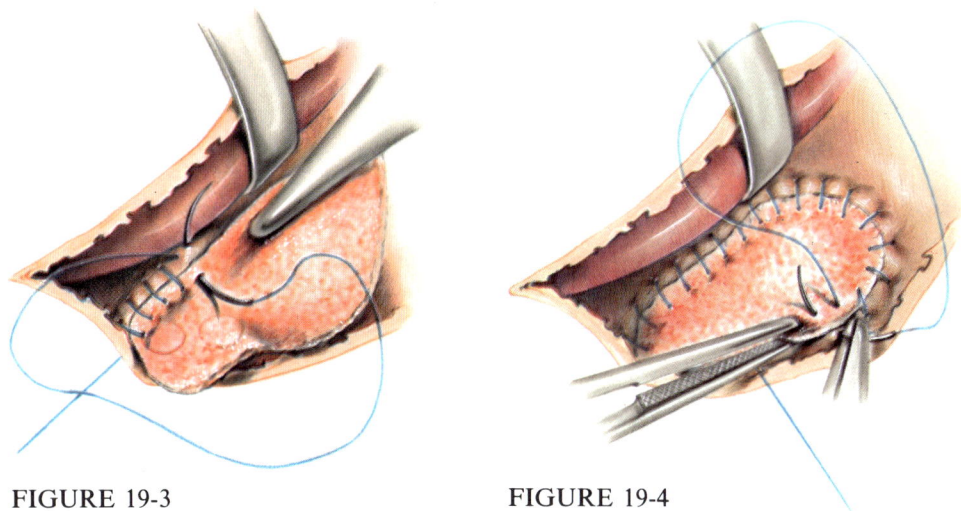

FIGURE 19-3   FIGURE 19-4

Results

Results vary, probably due to differences in surgical technique. Clark and colleagues[6] reported sinus node dysfunction in 70%, with 60% residual defects and 20% SVC obstruction in a group undergoing recatheterization. However, Trusler and co-workers[24] reported only minor electrocardiographic abnormalities, with normal sinus node recovery times, small residual defects in 22%, and SVC obstruction in 6%. Kyger and colleagues[15] report similarly good results. Excellent results are more likely to be achieved if repair is performed before age 15 years.

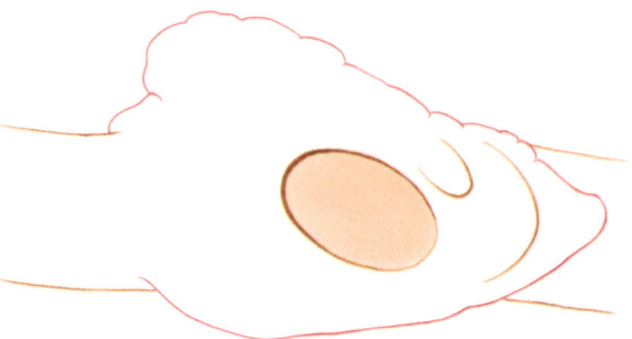

FIGURE 19-5

Ostium Secundum Defects

Surgical Anatomy
Secundum defects are located in the middle of the septum (Fig. 19-5). They may simply be large foramen ovale defects. They can extend toward the inferior vena cava (IVC) as well as posteriorly.[2] A large secundum defect may lack any ridge at the inferior caval junction.

Surgical Technique
The defect is exposed through a lateral atriotomy (Fig. 19-6) after institution of total bypass. The method of myocardial preservation is coronary perfusion through the aortic root at normothermia with electrically induced ventricular fibrillation.

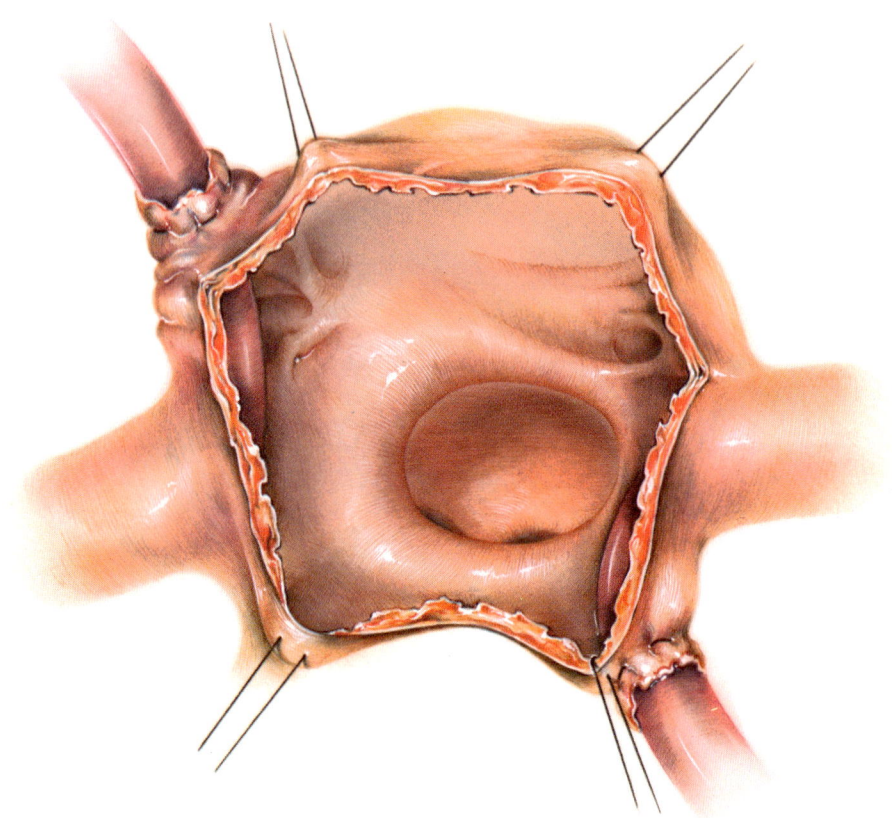

FIGURE 19-6

Many secundum defects can be closed primarily. The suture line is begun near the IVC orifice, frequently with a partial purse-string suture (Fig. 19-7). Such a suture closes the inferior margin of the defect securely and avoids the potential complication of creating a channel directing some IVC blood into the left atrium. The suture line is brought superiorly (Fig. 19-8), completing the closure. If the defect is large it is closed with a Dacron patch (Figs. 19-9, 19-10). Air is aspirated from the upper septum and the right superior pulmonary vein.

Results

Closure of secundum defects in children and young adults is associated with uniformly excellent results. Operative mortality is usually 0% and 90%–100% of patients are asymptomatic postoperatively.[7,26] Results are also good in adults, with usual relief of symptoms of dyspnea on exertion and fatigue.[10,12] In the elderly patient with congestive heart failure there is improvement, but not return to normal. Arrhythmias in adults are frequently unaffected by surgery.

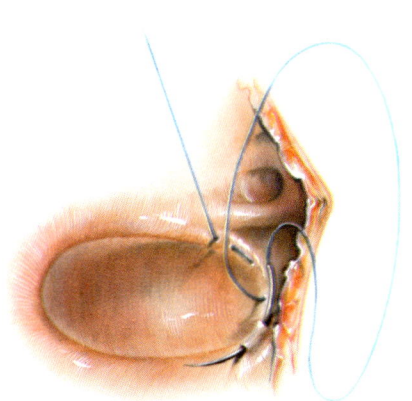
FIGURE 19-7

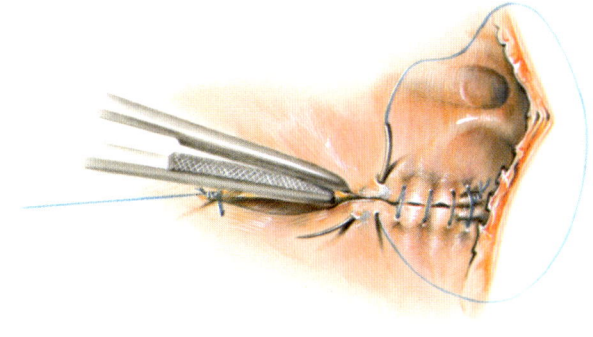
FIGURE 19-8

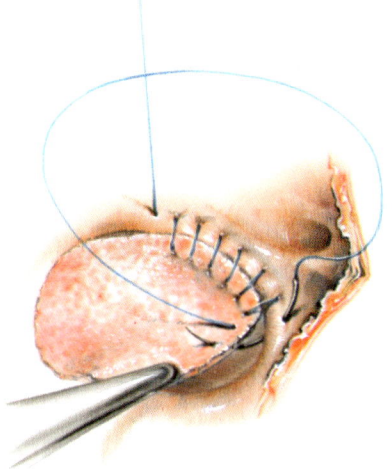
FIGURE 19-9

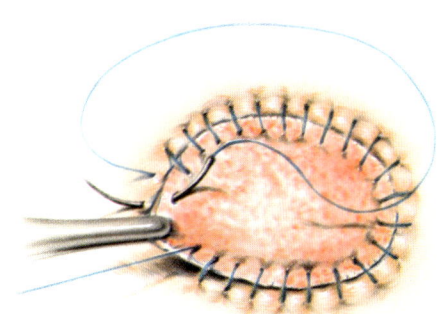
FIGURE 19-10

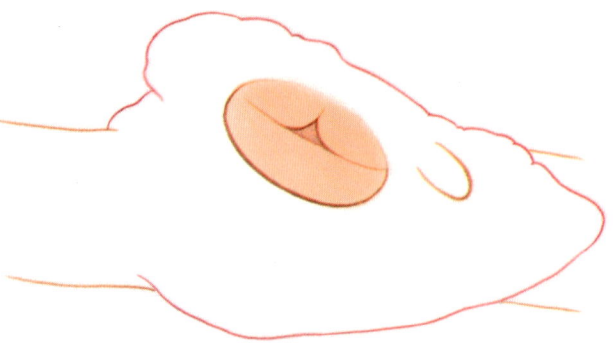

FIGURE 19-11

Ostium Primum Defect

Surgical Anatomy
Ostium primum defect is located in the inferior atrial septum and results from abnormal growth of the endocardial cushions (Fig. 19-11). A cleft in the anterior leaflet of the mitral valve is commonly present.

Surgical Technique
Myocardial preservation is usually cold crystalloid potassium cardioplegia, in order to obtain a completely bloodless field for precise suturing around the coronary sinus and enhanced exposure of the mitral valve.

Repair of the Mitral Valve
A suture is placed in the leading edge (free margin) of the anterior leaflet for alignment of closure of the cleft (Fig. 19-12). A fine running suture closes the cleft. Interrupted suture technique is also used. Pledgets are not used since they may stiffen the leaflet. Competence of the valve is checked by injecting cold saline through the valve with a large bulb syringe.

Closure of the Septal Defect
Precise suture placement near the base of the mitral valve and around the coronary sinus is necessary to avoid heart block. The inferior sutures are placed in the thickened tissue at the base of the anterior leaflet of the mitral valve[13] (Fig. 19-13). The suture line is carried toward the coronary sinus. At the transition point from the mitral leaflet to the atrial ridge near the coronary sinus, the sutures are placed right on the ridge or on the underside of the ridge. They should not be placed on the right atrial side of the ridge or near the coronary sinus, where injury to the atrioventricular node and bundle of His can occur.

The suture line is then carried laterally and superiorly to complete the closure (Fig. 19-14).

Results
Operative mortality for closure of ostium primum defects can approach 0%.[16] Approximately 80% of patients are asymptomatic. Late survival is excellent, with five-year survival of 95%.[17]

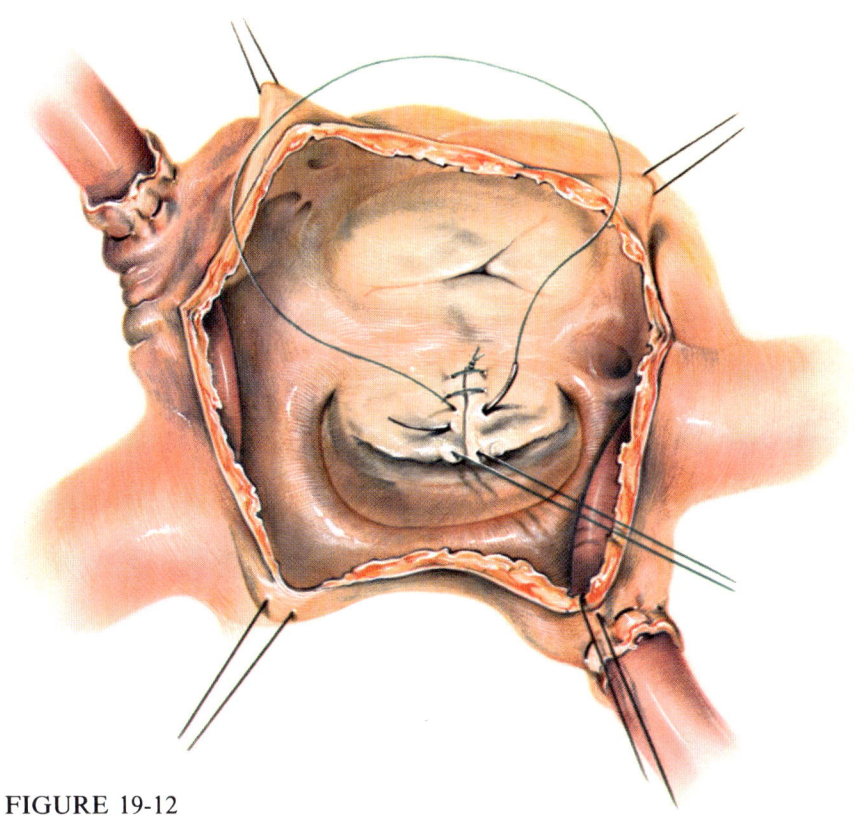

FIGURE 19-12

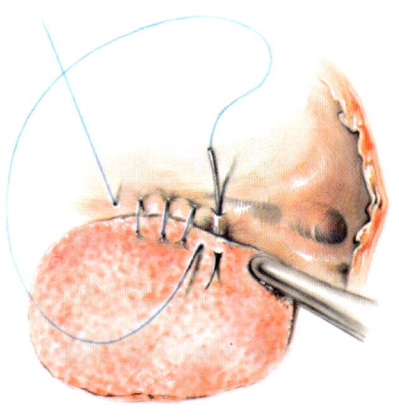

FIGURE 19-13

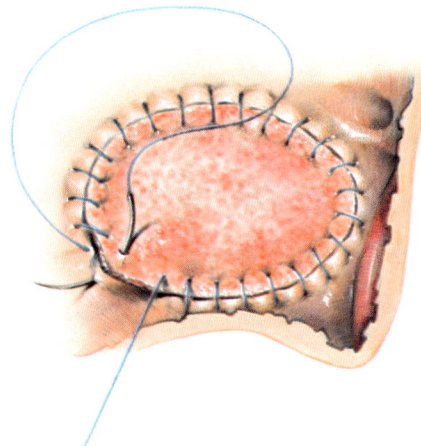

FIGURE 19-14

References

1. Beck W, Swan HJC, Burchell HB, Kirklin JW: Pulmonary vascular resistance after repair of atrial septal defects in patients with pulmonary hypertension. Circulation 22:938, 1960.
2. Bedford DE, Sellors TH, Sommerville W, Belcher JR, Besterman EMM: Atrial septal defect and its surgical treatment. Lancet 1:1255, 1957.
3. Braudo JL, Nadas AS, Rudolph AM, Neuhauser EBD: Atrial septal defects in children: a clinical study with special emphasis on indications for operative repair. Pediatrics 14:618, 1954.
4. Burrett JB, White PD: Large interauricular septal defect with particular reference to diagnosis and longevity. Am J Med Sci 209:355, 1945.
5. Campbell M, Neill C, Suzman S: Prognosis of atrial septal defect. Br Med J 1:1375, 1957.
6. Clark EB, Roland JMA, Varghese PJ, Neill CA, Haller JA: Should the sinus venosus type ASD be closed? A review of the atrial conduction defects and surgical results in twenty-eight children (abstr). Am J Cardiol 35:127, 1975.
7. Cooley DA: Results of surgical treatment of atrial septal defects. Am J Cardiol 6:605, 1960.
8. Davia JE, Cheitlin MD, Bedynek JL: Sinus venosus atrial septal defect: analysis of fifty cases. Am Heart J 85:177, 1973.
9. Dexter L: Atrial septal defect. Br Heart J 18:209, 1956.
10. Forgang K, Simonsen S, Andersen A, Efskind L: Atrial septal defect of secundum type in the middle-aged. Am Heart J 94:44, 1977.
11. Gibbon JH Jr: Application of a mechanical heart and lung apparatus to cardiac surgery. Minn Med 37:171, 1954.
12. Hairston P, Parker EF, Arrants JE, Bradham RR, Lee WH: The adult atrial septal defect. Ann Surg 179:799, 1974.
13. Hallman GL, Cooley DA: Surgical Treatment of Congenital Heart Disease, 2nd ed. Philadelphia, Lea & Febiger, 1975, p 85.
14. Kirklin JW, Ellis FH, Wood EH: Treatment of anomalous pulmonary venous connections in association with interatrial communications. Surgery 39:389, 1956.
15. Kyger ER III, Frazier OH, Cooley DA, Gillette PC, Reul GJ Jr, Sandiford FM, Wukasch DC: Sinus venosus atrial septal defect: early and late results following closure in 109 patients. Ann Thorac Surg 25:44, 1978.
16. Losay J, Rosenthal A, Castaneda AR, Bernhard WH, Nadas AS: Repair of atrial septal defect primum. J Thorac Cardiovasc Surg 75:248, 1978.
17. McMullan MH, McGoon DC, Wallace RB, Danielson GK, Weidman WH: Surgical treatment of partial atrioventricular canal. Arch Surg 107:705, 1973.
18. Phillips SJ, Okies JE, Henken D, Sunderland CO, Starr A: Complex of secundum atrial septal defect and congestive heart failure in infants. J Thorac Cardiovasc Surg 70:696, 1975.
19. Rahimtoola SH, Kirklin JW, Burchell HB: Atrial septal defect. Circulation 37(Suppl V):V-2, 1968.
20. Ross DN: The sinus venosus type of atrial septal defect. Guys Hosp Rep 105:376, 1956.
21. Schuster SR, Gross RE, Colodny AH: Surgical management of anomalous right pulmonary venous drainage to the superior vena cava, associated with superior marginal defect of the atrial septum. Surgery 51:805, 1962.
22. Somerville J: Ostium primum defect: factors causing deterioration in the natural history. Br Heart J 27:413, 1965.
23. Swan HJC, Zapata-Diaz J, Burchell HB, Wood EH: Pulmonary hypertension in congenital heart disease. Am J Med 16:12, 1954.
24. Trusler GA, Kazenelson G, Freedom RM, Williams WG, Rowe RD: Late results following repair of partial anomalous pulmonary venous connection with sinus venosus atrial septal defect. J Thorac Cardiovasc Surg 79:776, 1980.
25. Watson H (ed): Paediatric Cardiology, St Louis, CV Mosby Co, 1968.
26. Young D: Later results of closure of secundum atrial septal defect in children. Am J Cardiol 31:14, 1973.

Complete Atrioventricular Canal

20

The pioneering work in the 1960s by Rastelli and his colleagues[23,24] at the Mayo Clinic defined the anatomy of atrioventricular (AV) canal defects and developed a rational approach to surgical correction. Continued refinement of their basic principles has resulted in a surgical approach that is reproducible and predictable in its outcome.[9]

Indications for Surgery

The history of complete AV canal medically treated is associated with high mortality in the first months of life. Congestive heart failure secondary to large left-to-right shunting and/or AV valve incompetence results in death in 46% by 6 months of age, 65% by 12 months, and 85% by 24 months.[2] The development of pulmonary vascular disease is rapid and common. Newfeld and colleagues,[21] in a combined autopsy and lung biopsy study, found that two-thirds of patients had severe (Heath-Edwards[11] grade 3 or greater) pulmonary vascular disease by age 12 months.

The poor prognosis with medical treatment and the rapid development of pulmonary vascular disease have been the basis for recommending early total correction.[3,6,17] Correction before 2 years of age can be performed with an operative mortality of 25% or less—a mortality that appears much lower than that of nonsurgical treatment. It is our present policy to repair all complete AV canals by age 6 months or at the time of diagnosis.[1] Any patient in persistent congestive heart failure or failing to grow is repaired regardless of age or weight.

Pulmonary artery banding has been recommended as a preliminary surgical approach to AV canal in patients with a large ventricular shunt and minimal mitral insufficiency.[8] We do not agree with this approach, since banding is usually associated with a high mortality.[3,14] Banding may be indicated in very unusual situations, such as AV canal with multiple ventricular septal defects or in the case of underdevelopment of a ventricle.

Surgical Strategy

Operation in patients under 8 kg is performed using profound hypothermia and circulatory arrest (Chapter 5). In larger patients, standard bypass with systemic hypothermia is used. Cold crystalloid potassium cardioplegia is the method of myocardial preservation (Chapter 6).

Surgical Anatomy

Atrioventricular Defect
The septal defect in complete AV canal consists of an ostium primum type of atrial septal defect, a single common AV orifice, a deficiency in the upper ventricular septum, and a bare area on the crest of the ventricular septum. Between 30% and 50% of the expected surface area of the ventricular septum is usually missing.[7]

Atrioventricular Valves
The common AV orifice is bridged by anterior and posterior common leaflets that are not connected to each other. Rastelli and co-workers[23] based their classic classification on the configuration, relationships, and attachments of the anterior common leaflet, proposing three types: A, B, and C. Type A has an anterior common leaflet that is divided into two distinct portions, both of which are attached by chordae to the rim of the ventricular septum. In type B the anterior common leaflet is divided, but attached to chordae arising from an anomalous papillary muscle originating in the right ventricle from the ventricular septum. Type B is uncommon. In type C the anterior common leaflet is undivided and free floating, with essentially no chordal attachments to the septum. The posterior common leaflet varies widely in configuration, without any definite relationship to the anatomy of the anterior leaflet.[7,23]

The Rastelli classification is helpful, but is overly simple. There is enormous variability of the anterior and posterior leaflets that Rastelli's classification does not take into account.[3,5,22,27]

Conduction System
Knowledge of the conduction system anatomy is critical to prevent complete heart block as a complication of repair. Our knowledge of conduction system anatomy is based on the classic studies of Lev.[16]

The AV node is posteriorly displaced and is frequently directly adjacent to the coronary sinus ostium.[10] The bundle of His passes along the rim of the ventricular septum, dividing into the left and right bundle branches.

Ventricular Size and Dominance
Complete AV canal is usually associated with biventricular hypertrophy and increased volume of both ventricles.[12,26] However, hypoplasia of a ventricle may exist, with one ventricle being dominant, as described by Bharati and Lev.[4] The valve leaflets tend to be preferentially distributed into the larger ventricle. It is doubtful that such anatomy is suitable for correction. Echocardiography may be valuable in assessing ventricular size in complete AV canal.[19]

Surgical Technique

The atrium is opened and suspended. The anatomy of the atrium, ventricles, and atrioventricular valves is carefully and thoroughly inspected. Cold saline injected into the ventricles will float the valve leaflets and help to show their anatomy and relationships. This method is used to determine the location of incision of the common leaflets. A common location of incision of the anterior and posterior common leaflets is shown in Figure 20-1.

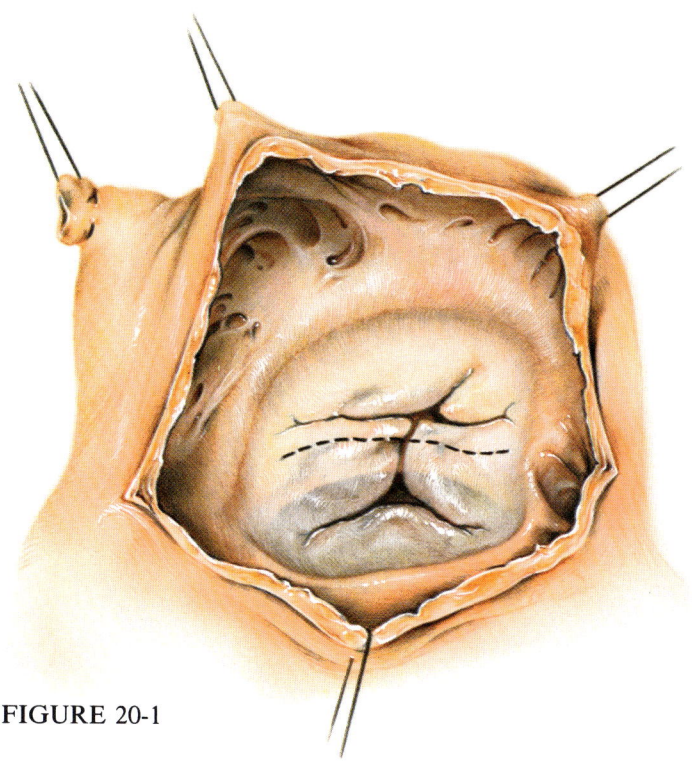

FIGURE 20-1

The anterior (Fig. 20-2) and posterior leaflets are divided as necessary. The most important principle of dividing the leaflets is to provide for an adequate amount of valve tissue on the left ventricular side. In special instances where a cleft is present in the anterior leaflet and division at the site of the cleft would leave deficient tissue, the cleft may be closed and the incision made farther to the right.[3]

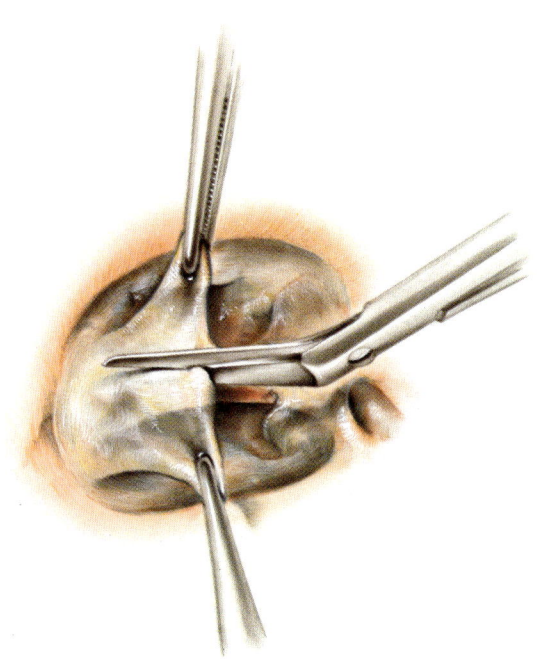

FIGURE 20-2

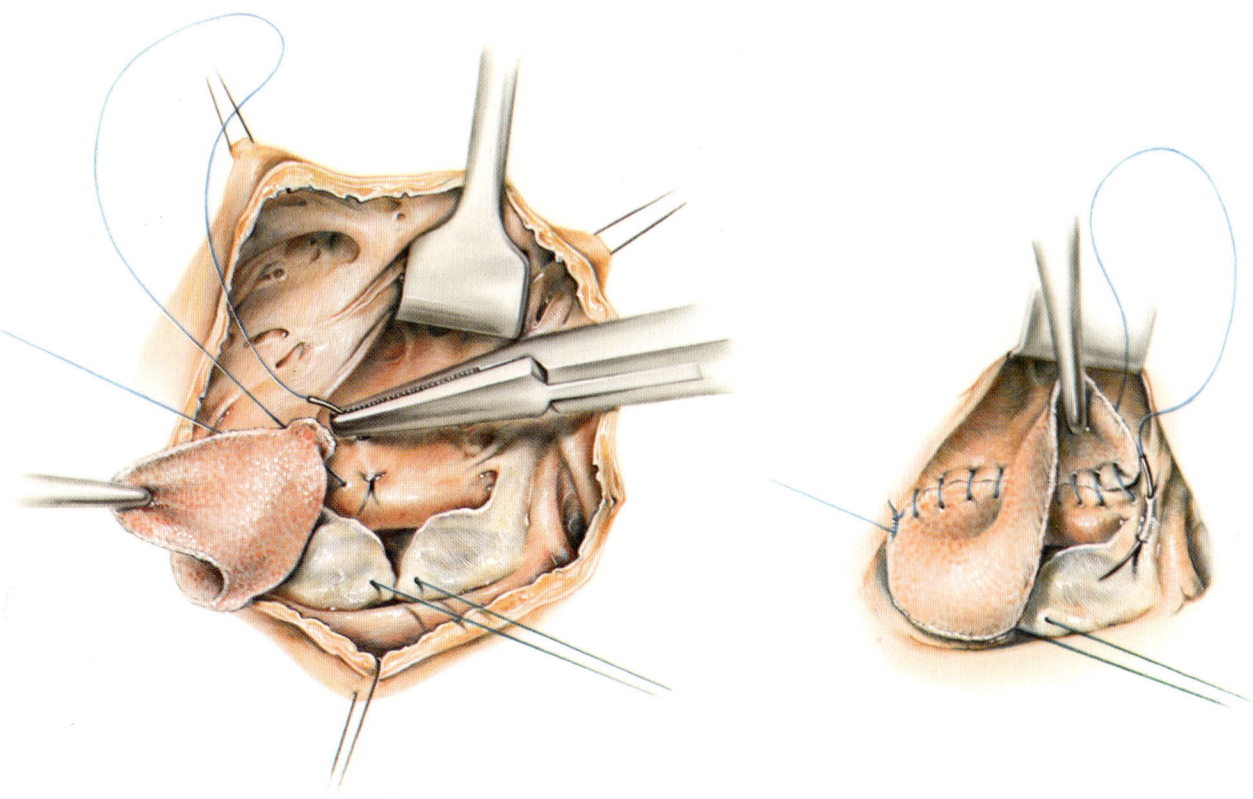

FIGURE 20-3   FIGURE 20-4

A single patch of Dacron double-velour is cut and carefully sized. Too large a patch will distort the AV valves by making the mitral anulus too large. A running suture of polypropylene is begun at the inferior portion of the ventricular defect and brought up, staying off the ridge on the right ventricular side in order to avoid injury to the conduction tissue (Fig. 20-3). As the suture line comes near the coronary sinus, superficial bites should be taken (Fig. 20-4) to avoid injury to the atrioventricular node.

The mitral valve is assessed to determine whether a bicuspid valve is to be constructed. This is determined by the size of the mural cusp. The valve is left tricuspid if rendering it bicuspid might make it stenotic.

For a bicuspid repair, the mitral components of the anterior and posterior common leaflets are joined, approximating the edges of the leaflets (Fig. 20-5). The height at which the valve is to be attached to the patch is then assessed. Short chordae connecting the ventricular septum may require cutting to release the leaflet for proper positioning (Fig. 20-6).

The proper height for attachment of the valve can be judged by a combination of factors, including the point at which the major chordae appear to be in proper alignment and the level of lateral attachment of the common leaflets. The midportion of the divided leaflets is usually attached to the patch at about the same level as their lateral attachments.

The leaflets are attached with a horizontal running mattress suture of fine polyester, placed well back from the cut edge of the leaflets, beginning with the mitral leaflet (Fig. 20-7) and working laterally (Figs. 20-8, 20-9).

Surgical Technique

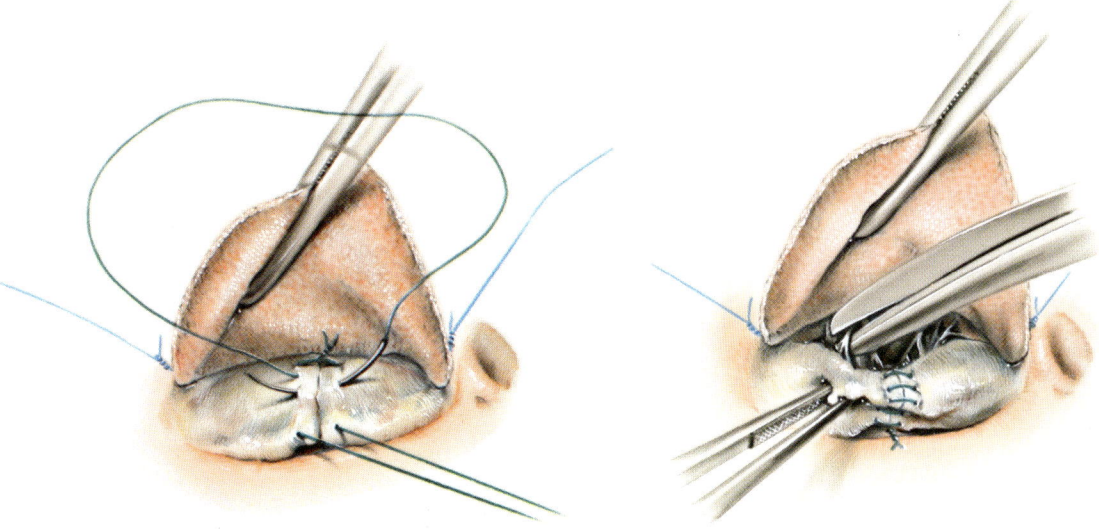

FIGURE 20-5

FIGURE 20-6

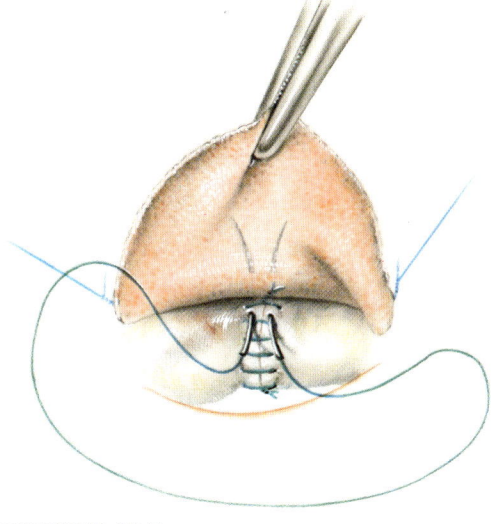

FIGURE 20-7

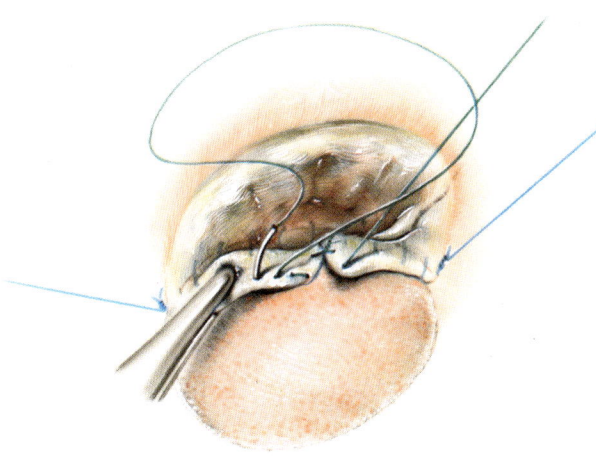

FIGURE 20-8

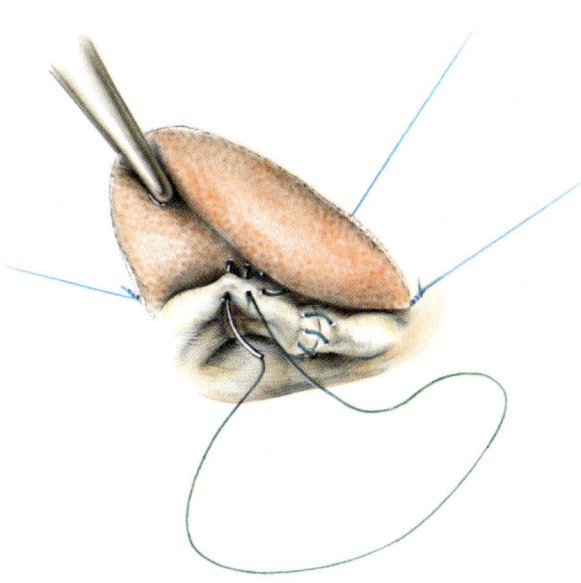

FIGURE 20-9

273

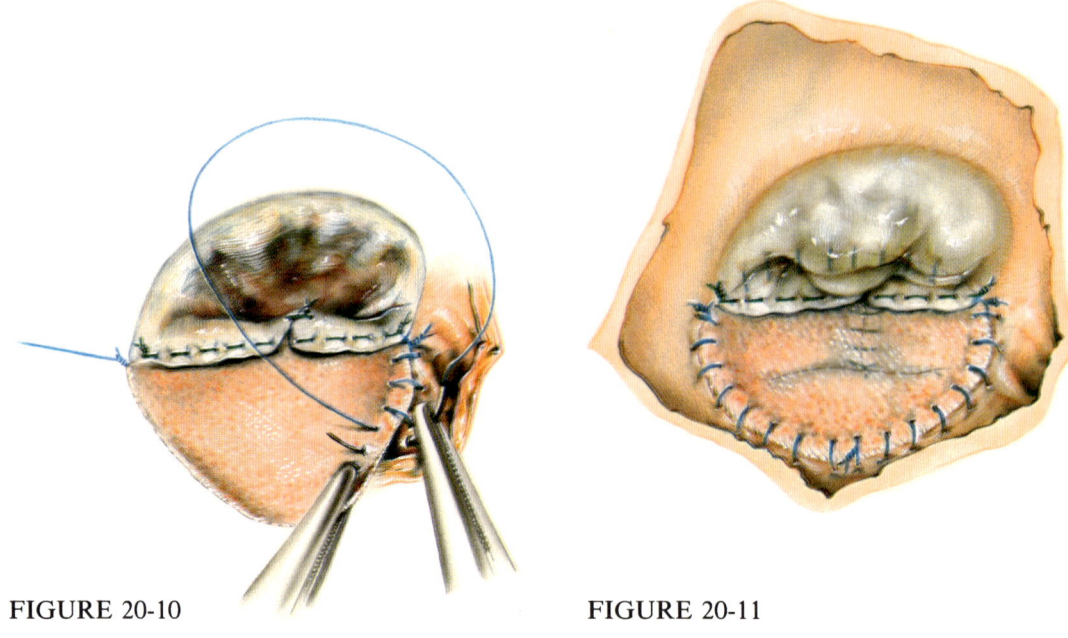

FIGURE 20-10 FIGURE 20-11

The valve is then checked for competence, and sutures are added as necessary to shorten the free edge of the leaflet, thereby increasing apposition of the leaflets.

The atrial portion of the repair is then completed (Figs. 20-10, 20-11). Alternative methods of repair, without dividing the anterior common leaflet and using separate patches, have been described, with satisfactory results.[15]

Results

Operative mortality in infancy can be as low as 20%–25%.[1,3,6,17,25] Two series of patients repaired during childhood have been reported with 0% operative mortality.[13,20]

Functional and hemodynamic results are good. Hemodynamically significant mitral regurgitation is rare.[3,6,13] Elevated pulmonary vascular resistance usually returns to normal.[13]

Late survival is excellent.[18] Berger and colleagues[3] report a five-year survival rate of 91% among hospital survivors. A recent series at the University of Oregon, of patients undergoing repair during the first six months of life, has had no late deaths (follow-up 2–20 months).[1]

References

1. Abbruzzese PA, Kirby WC, Sunderland CO, Starr A: Primary repair of complete A-V canal during the first 6 months of life. Unpublished data.
2. Berger TJ, Blackstone EH, Kirklin JW, Bargeron LM, Hazelrig JB, Turner ME: Survival and probability of cure without and with operation in complete atrioventricular canal. Ann Thorac Surg 27:104, 1979.
3. Berger TJ, Kirklin JW, Blackstone EH, Pacifico AD, Kouchoukos NT: Primary repair of complete atrioventricular canal in patients less than 2 years old. Am J Cardiol 41:906, 1978.
4. Bharati S, Lev M: The spectrum of common atrioventricular orifice (canal). Am Heart J 86:553, 1973.
5. Bharati S, Lev M, McAllister HA, Kirklin JW: Surgical anatomy of the atrioventricular valve in the intermediate type of common atrioventricular orifice. J Thorac Cardiovasc Surg 79:884, 1980.

6. Culpepper W, Kolff J, Chung-Yuan L, Vitullo D, Lamberti D, Lamberti J, Arcilla RA, Replogle R: Complete common atrioventricular canal in infancy—surgical repair and postoperative hemodynamics. Circulation 58:550, 1978.
7. Ebert P, Goor DA: Complete atrioventricular canal malformation: further clarification of the anatomy of the common leaflet and its relationship to the VSD in surgical correction. Ann Thorac Surg 25:134, 1978.
8. Epstein ML, Moller JH, Amplatz K, Nicoloff DM: Pulmonary artery banding in infants with complete atrioventricular canal. J Thorac Cardiovasc Surg 78:28, 1979.
9. Feldt RH (ed): Atrioventricular Canal Defects. Philadelphia, London, Toronto, WB Saunders Co, 1976.
10. Feldt RH, DuShane JW, Titus JL: The atrioventricular conduction system in persistent common atrioventricular canal defect: correlations with the electrocardiogram. Circulation 42:437, 1970.
11. Heath D, Edwards JE: Pathology of hypertensive vascular disease: a description of six grades of structural changes in the pulmonary arteries with special reference to congenital cardiac septal defects. Circulation 43:533, 1958.
12. Jarmakani JM, George B, Wheeler J: Ventricular volume characteristics in infants and children with endocardial cushion defects. Circulation 58:153, 1978.
13. Kahn DR, Levy J, France NE, Chung KJ, Dacumos GD: Recent results after repair of atrioventricular canal. J Thorac Cardiovasc Surg 73:413, 1977.
14. Kirklin JW, Blackstone EH: Management of the infant with complete atrioventricular canal. J Thorac Cardiovasc Surg 78:32, 1979.
15. Kirklin JW, Chung G, Pacifico AD, Blackstone EH, Bargeron LM: The repair of A-V canal defects in the first 3 months of life. Presented at Bergamo, Italy, 1980.
16. Lev M: The architecture of the conduction system in congenital heart disease. I. Common atrioventricular orifice. Arch Pathol 65:174, 1958.
17. Mair DD, McGoon DC: Surgical correction of atrioventricular canal during the first year of life. Am J Cardiol 40:66, 1977.
18. McMullan MH, Wallace RB, Weidman WH, McGoon DC: Surgical treatment of complete atrioventricular canal. Surgery 72:905, 1972.
19. Mehta S, Hirschfield S, Riggs T, Liebman J: Echocardiographic estimation of ventricular hypoplasia in complete atrioventricular canal. Circulation 59:888, 1979.
20. Mills ML, Ochsner JL, King TD: Correction of Type C complete atrioventricular canal: surgical considerations. J Thorac Cardiovasc Surg 71:20, 1976.
21. Newfeld EA, Sher M, Paul MH, Nikaidoh H: Pulmonary vascular disease in complete atrioventricular canal defect. Am J Cardiol 39:721, 1977.
22. Piccoli GP, Wilkinson JL, Macartney FJ, Gerlis LM, Anderson RH: Morphology and classification of complete atrioventricular defects. Br Heart J 42:633, 1979.
23. Rastelli G, Kirklin JW, Titus JL: Anatomic observations on complete form of persistent common atrioventricular canal with special reference to atrioventricular valves. Mayo Clin Proc 41:296, 1966.
24. Rastelli GC, Ongley PA, Kirklin JW, McGoon DC: Surgical repair of the complete form of persistent common atrioventricular canal. J Thorac Cardiovasc Surg 55:299, 1968.
25. Stewart S, Harris P, Manning J: Complete endocardial cushion defect: operative technique and results. J Thorac Cardiovasc Surg 78:914, 1979.
26. Thanopoulos BD, Fisher EA, DuBrow IW, Hastreiter AR: Right and left ventricular volume characteristics in common atrioventricular canal. Circulation 57:991, 1978.
27. Ugarte M, de Salamanca FE, Quero M: Endocardial cushion defects: an anatomical study of 54 specimens. Br Heart J 38:674, 1976.

21 Ventricular Septal Defects

Isolated ventricular septal defect (VSD) is the most common congenital cardiac defect, with an incidence of approximately 2 per 1000 live births.[17] Isolated VSD accounts for 25% of all congenital heart disease.[21] The wide range of physiology and natural history of VSDs necessitates careful consideration of operative indications and timing. Understanding of the anatomic variations and applicable surgical techniques is necessary to achieve the excellent results that are possible today.

Indications for Surgery

The indications for surgery of VSDs are influenced by the wide variation in natural history. Some defects close or decrease in size early in life. Approximately one-third of all defects will spontaneously close, and another third will become smaller during the first two years of life.[16,17,21,31] Other defects follow a benign course for many years. However, some follow a course of congestive heart failure (CHF), failure to thrive, recurrent pulmonary infections, or development of pulmonary vascular disease. Timely intervention with surgical treatment is necessary in the latter group to prevent development of irreversible pulmonary vascular disease or death secondary to CHF.

Infants with clinically small defects should be followed. Infants with CHF should have medical treatment instituted and the response assessed. Those who have persistence of CHF or intractable respiratory distress should have early catheterization and surgery.[22] Those with good response to medical treatment should be followed, at least until age six months, to determine whether there is any evidence of spontaneous closure or decrease in the size of the defect. It must be remembered that clinical evidence of decreasing left-to-right shunt may also be caused by development of infundibular stenosis or rising pulmonary vascular resistance (PVR). Contrast echocardiography may be useful for following these patients.[39]

If evidence of a large shunt persists or rise in pulmonary artery pressure is suggested, catheterization should be performed. Patients with shunts less than 2:1 and pulmonary artery pressure less than one-third systemic pressure should be managed conservatively. Patients with shunts over 2:1 must be carefully considered for surgery, taking into account their overall clinical status and pulmonary vascular resistance.

Blackstone, Kirklin, and colleagues[5] have performed a careful study of the optimal age related to late results in elective repair of large ventricular septal defects. They found that the age at operation, the preoperative pulmonary vascular resistance, and preoperative pulmonary artery pressure were directly related to the mean pulmonary artery pressure five or more years later. For such elective or semielective patients they recommend waiting until about 2 years of age if the PVR is low (less than 4 units/m^2). If the PVR is moderately elevated (8 units/m^2) operation should be done at about 6 months of age, hopefully to avoid established pulmonary vascular disease. If PVR is markedly elevated (12 units/m^2), but pulmonary blood flow is 1.3 or more times systemic blood flow, operation should be done promptly, even before 6 months of age. We agree with these recommendations for elective surgery. As stated earlier, urgent operation is recommended regardless of age or size for infants who are severely symptomatic, have serious growth retardation, or have intractable CHF.

Older children or adults with VSD should undergo closure if a pulmonary-to-systemic flow ratio of 2:1 or more is present.[34] Patients with a smaller shunt should also be considered for surgery under some circumstances, such as recurrent bacterial endocarditis, fear of progressive aortic insufficiency with supracristal defects, or where there is a disparity between symptoms and calculated shunt.

Choice of Operation

The high mortality during the 1950s and early 1960s of open repair of VSD in infancy prompted the adoption of two-stage management, consisting of initial palliation by pulmonary artery banding[32] followed by later open closure of the VSD and debanding of the pulmonary artery.[14,40] This approach has generally fallen from use over the past decade owing to the excellent results that can now be achieved by primary total correction, regardless of age or size.

The cumulative mortality of the two-stage approach is 20%–30% in most series.[9,29] This mortality greatly exceeds the 5% or lower mortality that can be achieved by primary total correction.[1,2,46] Pulmonary artery banding for isolated VSD has become obsolete.[13] However, in unusual situations, such as multiple VSDs, we continue to employ pulmonary artery banding on a selective basis.

Surgical Strategy

Method of Cardiopulmonary Bypass
The technique of profound hypothermia and circulatory arrest is used for most infants weighing less than 8 kg. In all other patients standard cardiopulmonary bypass with moderate systemic hypothermia is used (Chapter 5).

Myocardial Preservation
Cold potassium crystalloid cardioplegia is the method in all cases (Chapter 6).

Management of Aortic Insufficiency
The association of aortic insufficiency (AI) with VSD is rare, with a reported incidence of 2%–4%.[35,37] The AI is most often caused by prolapse of the right coronary cusp.[10,42,56] Hypotheses regarding causation of the AI include trauma to the valve by the surge of blood through the VSD[48] and a deficiency in anatomic structures supporting the aortic valve anulus and the sinus of Valsalva.

Many approaches to management of aortic insufficiency have been recommended, from doing nothing to the valve to replacement of the valve. Although minimal AI may be corrected by simply closing the VSD, moderate to severe AI requires valvuloplasty or valve replacement.

Many techniques of valvuloplasty have been described, most involving suspension and/or shortening of the free margin of the prolapsing leaflet.[18,33,41,43,44,53] Because of the small number of patients in any one series, it is impossible to determine whether any specific technique of valvuloplasty is clearly superior.[43] Failure of valvuloplasty appears to be more likely if the AI is severe and of long duration. Valve replacement has been recommended in adults with VSD and associated AI.[37]

Surgical Anatomy

Defect Location (Fig. 21-1)

The classic studies of Becu[3] and Kirklin[23] formed the basis for a widely used classification of VSDs. This classification utilizes the major anatomic landmarks of the interior of the right ventricle as reference points, the most important being the crista supraventricularis. Other classifications[28] use the trabecula septomarginalis, as defined by Tandler,[47] as the main reference point.

Becu and Kirklin divide the right ventricle into an inflow tract and an outflow tract. The outflow tract is that part which lies between the pulmonary valve above and the tricuspid valve below. The four major anatomic landmarks of the outflow tract of the right ventricle are the tricuspid ring, the papillary

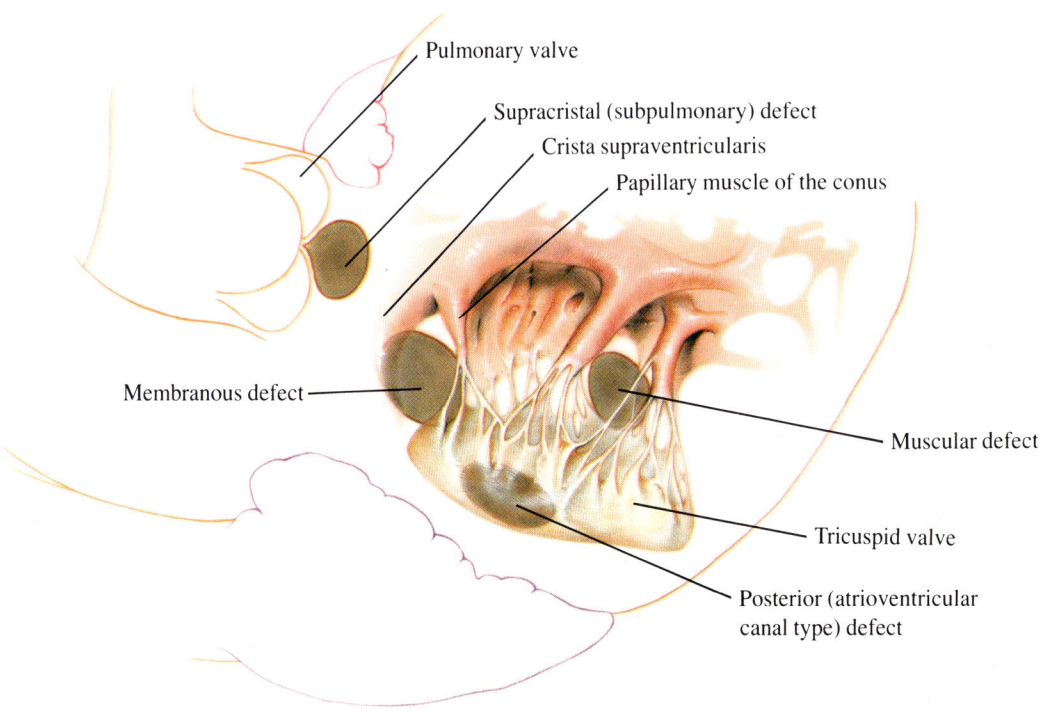

FIGURE 21-1

muscle of the conus, the crista supraventricularis, and the anulus fibrosus of the pulmonary valve. Most of the outflow tract of the right ventricle and the pulmonary valve lies more cephalad and anterior than the left ventricular outflow tract and aortic valve, so the crista supraventricularis overlies a portion of the root of the aorta. These anatomic characteristics explain the frequent intimate relationship of VSDs in the right ventricular outflow tract with portions of the aortic valve.

The most common location of VSDs is just inferior to the crista supraventricularis in the region of the membranous septum—the "membranous defect."[14,23,28] These defects usually involve more than just absence of membranous septum and have variable amounts of muscular septal deficiency. Membranous defects account for approximately 75%–85% of VSDs. They have also been termed subaortic or conoventricular.[36] From the left ventricular side they are under the right coronary cusp and noncoronary cusp.

The other location of defects in the right ventricular outflow tract is above the crista supraventricularis, just below the pulmonary valve—"supracristal type." The anulus fibrosus of the pulmonary valve usually forms the upper border of these defects. From the left ventricular side the supracristal defect is under the left coronary cusp.

Defects in the inflow are either posterior under the septal leaflet or in the midportion or apical portion of the muscular septum. Defects high and posterior have been termed "atrioventricular canal type," but we prefer "posterior," since this terminology is less confusing. From the left ventricular side, posterior defects are between the posteromedial papillary muscle and the mitral valve.

The last major type of defect is "muscular," lying either in the midportion of the septum or near the apex.[57] Muscular defects may be multiple.

Conduction System

Knowledge of the anatomy of the conduction system and its relationship to the various types of defects is important to avoid surgical injury to conduction tissue.[26]

In the normal heart the major portion of the atrioventricular (AV) node is located in the lower right atrium, to the left of the coronary sinus.[38,49,52] The terminal portion of the AV node is in the atrial septum at its attachment to the central fibrous body. The central fibrous body is at the confluence of the AV valves, the atrial septum, membranous ventricular septum, and aortic valve ring.

The bundle of His begins as a continuation of the AV node at the right fibrous trigone and pierces the membranous ventricular septum or skirts the septum posteriorly to enter the summit of the muscular ventricular septum, where it gives off multiple left branches. The bundle of His continues as the right bundle branch on the right side of the muscular septum.

The location of the VSD usually determines the relationship of the bundle of His and bundle branches.[25,30,50,51] In the most common type of VSD, the membranous, the conduction tissue is usually on the posterior-inferior aspect of the defect and may be on the rim or on the left or right side of the rim. In the posterior defects the conduction tissue may pass in the superior aspect of the defect.[30] The conduction tissue is usually distant from supracristal defects and muscular defects.

Milo[30] and Lincoln[28] have recommended that the apex of the triangle of Koch[24] be used as the guide to the location of the conduction tissue. The "base" of the triangle is the coronary sinus. The apex of the triangle is where the tendon of Todaro (a rim of tissue from the top of the coronary sinus to

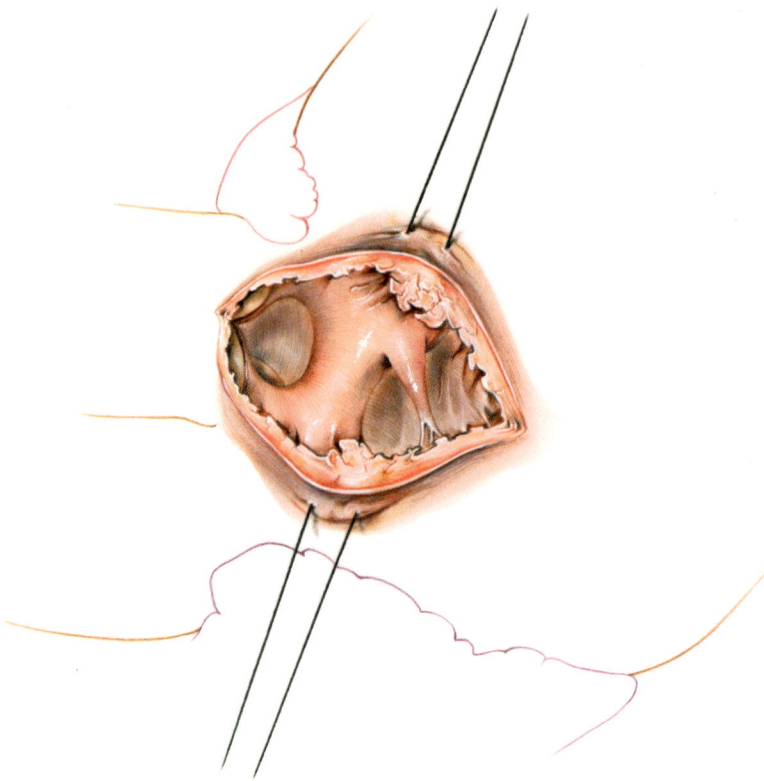

FIGURE 21-2

the septal leaflet) meets the attachment of the septal leaflet. As examined from the right atrium, the membranous defects will generally be to the left of this apex; the posterior defects will be to the right. Sutures can therefore be placed in a manner to avoid the conduction tissue.

Surgical Technique

A number of approaches to repair of VSDs have been described. In addition to the usual right atrial or right ventricular approaches, closure through the aortic valve[12,15] or pulmonary valve[19] has also been described. Our standard approach to supracristal defects is via right ventriculotomy; to membranous, posterior, and some muscular defects is via the right atrium; and to apical defects is via left ventriculotomy.

Surgical Technique

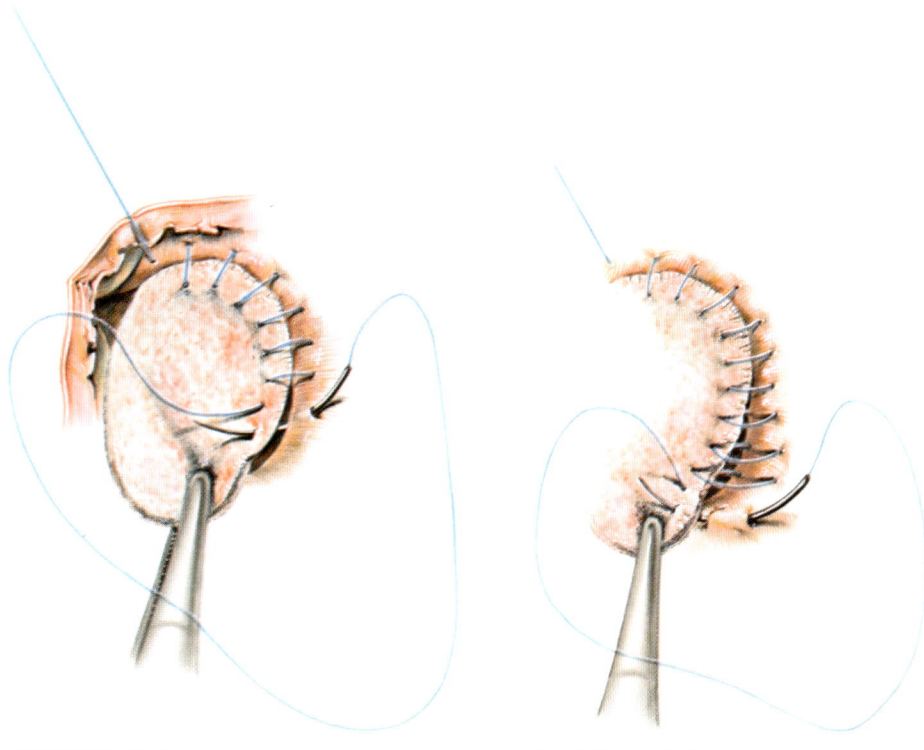

FIGURE 21-3

FIGURE 21-4

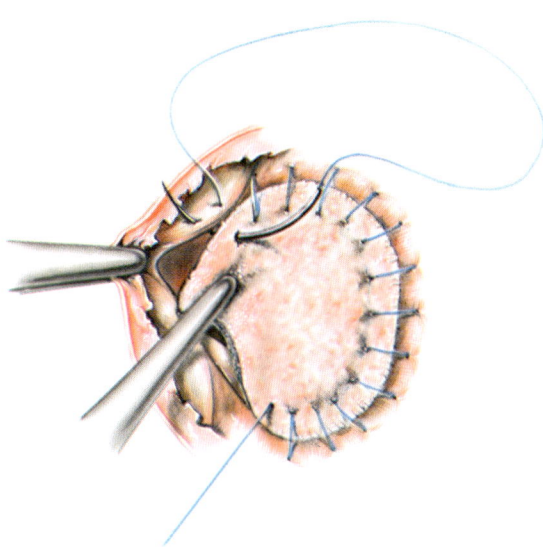

FIGURE 21-5

Supracristal Type

A short vertical ventriculotomy is made below the pulmonary valve, exposing the defect (Fig. 21-2). A patch of Dacron is cut to appropriate size. The suture line of polypropylene is begun at the far rim and brought around the lower rim (Figs. 21-3, 21-4). The upper border is then sutured, with stitches being taken near or into the anulus of the pulmonary valve (Fig. 21-5). Special care must be taken to avoid injuring the pulmonary valve leaflets or underlying aortic valve. Rarely, supracristal defects can be closed through the right atrium. Exploration through the atrium should always precede ventriculotomy.

281

Membranous Type

Transatrial closure was suggested during the early years of VSD surgery,[8] particularly in the case of defects with high pulmonary vascular resistance,[4,7,20,27] since this approach avoided the deleterious hemodynamic effects of a right ventriculotomy.[45] With increasing experience and especially with the improved exposure provided by the flaccid heart of cold cardioplegic arrest, the atrial approach has become our choice and can be used for the great majority of defects.

The atrium is opened from below the appendage to near the inferior caval junction. A suture can be placed in the anterior leaflet of the tricuspid valve to help expose the defect (Fig. 21-6). Rarely, one or two chordae to the septal leaflet must be cut to obtain good exposure. Although small defects may be closed by simple suture, most defects are closed using a Dacron patch. The suture line of polypropylene is begun on the right side of the inferior rim and carried in a counterclockwise direction to penetrate the septal leaflet.

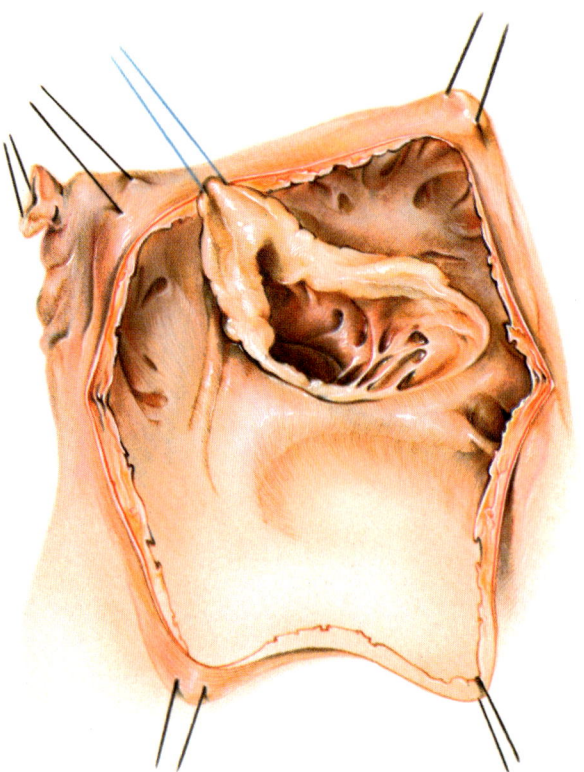

FIGURE 21-6

The other arm is carried clockwise (Fig. 21-7) and brought around (Fig. 21-8). The upper portion of the patch is then sutured to the base of the septal leaflet (*not* through the anulus) with pledgets or a single strip of Teflon buttressing the repair on the atrial side of the leaflet (Fig. 21-9). Horizontal mattress sutures are used and are tied after they have all been placed.

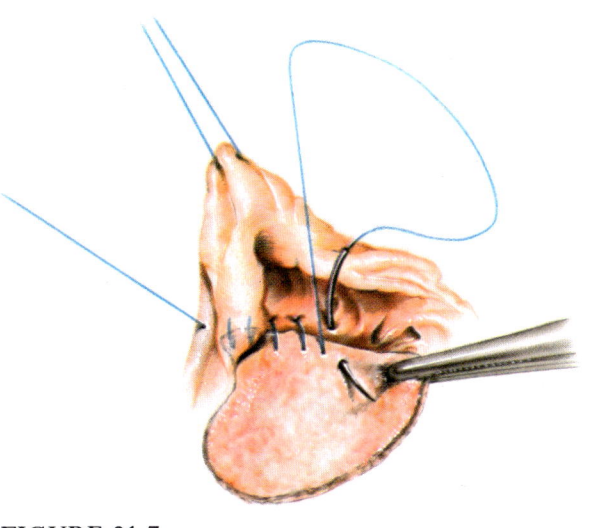

FIGURE 21-7

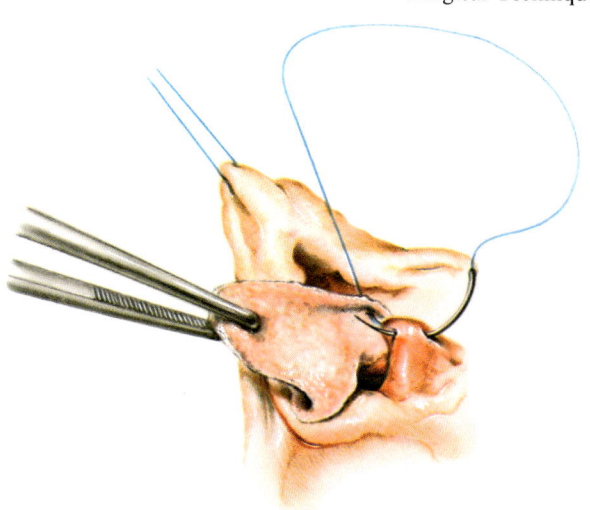

FIGURE 21-8

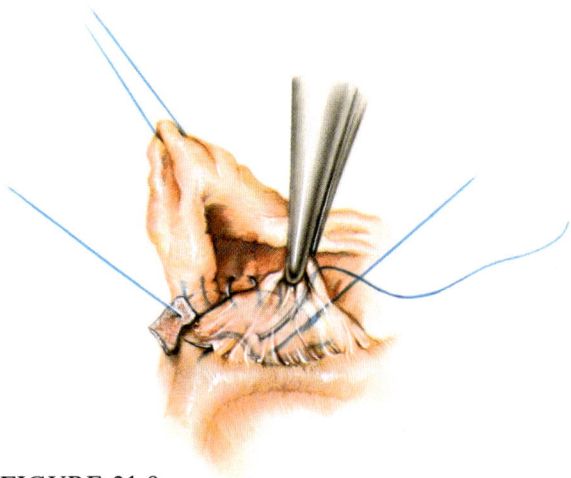

FIGURE 21-9

Posterior Defects

Posterior defects may be overlaid by papillary muscles and chordae (Fig. 21-10). Many are suitable for primary repair with buttressed horizontal mat-

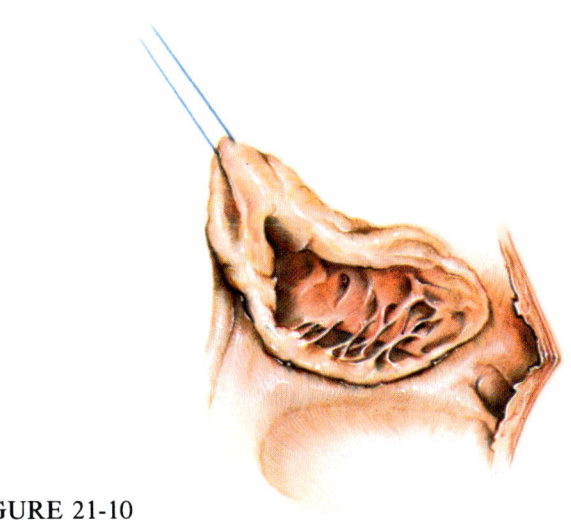

FIGURE 21-10

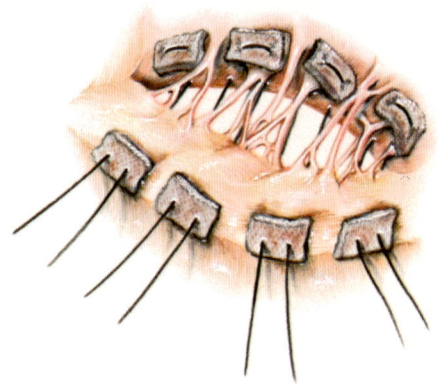

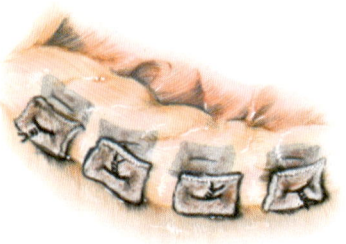

FIGURE 21-12

FIGURE 21-11

tress sutures. The sutures are placed through the right side of the defect and the base of the septal leaflet (Fig. 21-11) and tied (Fig. 21-12).

Muscular Defects

Most defects in the midportion of the septum can be exposed through the tricuspid valve (Fig. 21-13) and closed primarily or with a patch (Fig. 21-14). If the defect is toward the apex, a limited left ventriculotomy is made between the distal left anterior descending and diagonal coronary arteries, and the defect is closed from the left ventricular side.[41]

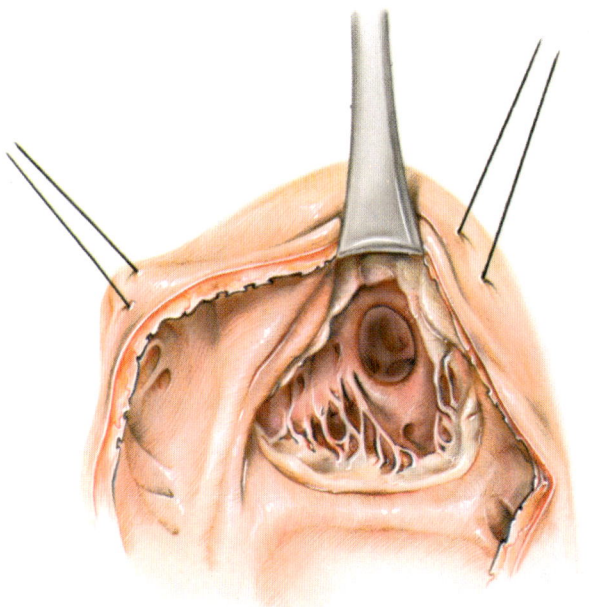

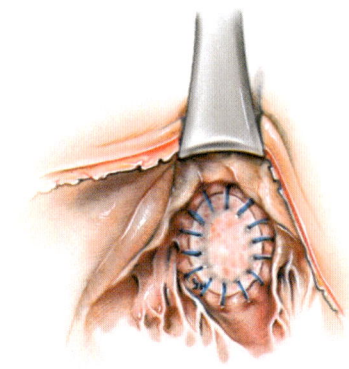

FIGURE 21-14

FIGURE 21-13

Pulmonary Artery Banding

In the case of normally related great arteries, a left lateral thoracotomy is made through the fourth interspace. The pericardium is incised longitudinally anterior to the phrenic nerve and suspended. The plane between the pulmonary artery and aorta is opened, and a right angle is passed around the pulmonary artery. A silicone-coated strip of Teflon is then brought around the pulmonary artery.

There are several methods of determining the degree of banding, including pressure measurements and predetermination of band circumference. Pressure measurement has not been completely reliable as a means of evaluating adequacy of a pulmonary artery band. This may be due to the variations in pulmonary vascular resistance and systemic vascular resistance during and after pulmonary artery banding.[55] An alternate method of determining the proper degree of banding is the use of a premarked measured band, with the size of the band being calculated from the patient's body weight.[54] We have used the technique of a premarked measured band in a small number of cases and find it to be satisfactory. Any method of assessment must, of course, take into account the immediate clinical effect of the band, with appropriate adjustments being made as necessary.

Results

Operative mortality for closure of VSD during infancy can be as low as 2%–4%.[1,2,11,46] Late survival is excellent and growth usually returns to normal.[6,36] Pulmonary artery pressure and pulmonary vascular resistance are usually normal one year postoperatively.[36] Closure of VSD in childhood can be associated with operative mortality as low as 0% and excellent late survival.[5]

References

1. Agosti J, Chiarello L, Wagner H, Subramanian S: Intracardiac repair of isolated ventricular septal defects below two years of age. J Cardiovasc Surg 17:147, 1976.
2. Barratt-Boyes BG, Neutze JM, Clarkson PM, Shardey GC, Brandt PWT: Repair of ventricular septal defect in the first two years of life using profound hypothermia–circulatory arrest techniques. Ann Surg 184:376, 1976.
3. Becu LM, Fontana RS, DuShane JW, Kirklin JW, Burchell HB, Edwards JE: Anatomic and pathologic studies in ventricular septal defect. Circulation 14:349, 1956.
4. Bjork VO: The transatrial approach to ventricular septal defect. J Thorac Cardiovasc Surg 47:178, 1964.
5. Blackstone EH, Kirklin JW, Bradley EL, DuShane JW, Appelbaum A: Optimal age and results in repair of large ventricular septal defects. J Thorac Cardiovasc Surg 72:661, 1976.
6. Cartmill TB, DuShane JW, McGoon DC, Kirklin JW: Results of repair of ventricular septal defect. J Thorac Cardiovasc Surg 52:486, 1966.
7. Castaneda AR, Zamora R, Nicoloff DM, Moller JH, Hunt CE, Lucas RV: High-pressure, high-resistance ventricular septal defect. Ann Thorac Surg 12:29, 1971.
8. Cooley DA, Belmonte BA, DeBakey ME, Latson JR: Temporary extracorporeal circulation in the surgical treatment of cardiac and aortic disease. Ann Surg 145:898, 1957.
9. Dooley KJ, Parisi-Buckley L, Fyler DC, Nadas AS: Results of pulmonary arterial banding in infancy: survey of 5 years' experience in the New England Regional Infant Cardiac Program. Am J Cardiol 36:484, 1975.
10. Ellis FH, Ongley PA, Kirklin JW: Ventricular septal defect with aortic valvular incompetence. Surgical considerations. Circulation 27:789, 1963.
11. Fisher RD, Faulkner SL, Sell CG, Graham TP Jr, Bender HW Jr: Operative closure of isolated defects of the ventricular septum: planned delay. Ann Thorac Surg 26:351, 1978.

12. Galioto FM Jr, Cooley DA, El-Said G, Mullin CE, Sandiford FM: Closure of ventricular septal defect through the aortic valve. Chest 64:683, 1973.
13. Griepp E, French JW, Shumway NE, Baum D: Is pulmonary artery banding for ventricular septal defects obsolete? Circulation 49,50(Suppl II):II–14, 1974.
14. Hallman GL, Cooley DA, Bloodwell RD: Two-stage surgical treatment of ventricular septal defect: results of pulmonary artery banding in infants and subsequent open-heart repair. J Thorac Cardiovasc Surg 52:476, 1966.
15. Harlan BJ, Cooley DA: Transaortic repair of double-outlet right ventricle with situs inversus, l-loop, l-malposition (I,L,L), subaortic ventricular septal defect, and associated anomalies. J Thorac Cardiovasc Surg 72:547, 1976.
16. Hoffman JIE: Natural history of congenital heart disease. Circulation 37:97, 1968.
17. Hoffman JIE, Rudolph AM: Natural history of ventricular septal defect in infancy. Am J Cardiol 16:634, 1965.
18. Kawashima Y, Danno M, Shimizu Y, Matsuda H, Miyamoto T, Fujita T, Kozuka T, Manabe H: Ventricular septal defect associated with aortic insufficiency. Anatomic classification and method of operation. Circulation 47:1057, 1973.
19. Kawashima Y, Fujita T, Mori T, Ihara K, Manabe H: Transpulmonary arterial closure of ventricular septal defect. J Thorac Cardiovasc Surg 74:191, 1977.
20. Kay JH, Anderson RM, Tolentino P, Dykstra P, Shapiro MJ, Meihaus JE, Magidson O: The surgical repair of high pressure ventricular septal defect through the right atrium. Surgery 48:65, 1960.
21. Keith JD, Rose V, Collins G, Kidd BSL: Ventricular septal defect: incidence, morbidity, and mortality in various age groups. Br Heart J 33:81, 1971 (Suppl).
22. Kirklin JW, DuShane JW: Repair of ventricular septal defect in infancy. Pediatrics 27:961, 1961.
23. Kirklin JW, Harshbarger HG, Donald DE, Edwards JE: Surgical correction of ventricular septal defect: anatomic and technical considerations. J Thorac Surg 33:45, 1957.
24. Koch W: Weitere mitteilungen uber den Sinusknoten des Herzens. Verh Dtsch Ges Pathol 13:85, 1909.
25. Lev M: The architecture of the conduction system in congenital heart disease. III. Ventricular septal defect. Arch Pathol 70:529, 1970.
26. Lev M, Fell EH, Arcilla R, Weinberg MH: Surgical injury to the conduction system in ventricular septal defect. Am J Cardiol 14:464, 1964.
27. Lillehei CW, Levy MJ, Adams P, Anderson RC: High-pressure ventricular septal defects. JAMA 188:949, 1964.
28. Lincoln C, Jamieson S, Joseph M, Shinebourne E, Anderson RH: Transatrial repair of ventricular septal defects with reference to their anatomic classification. J Thorac Cardiovasc Surg 74:183, 1977.
29. McNicholas KW, Bowman FO Jr, Hayes CJ, Edie RN, Malm JR: Surgical management of ventricular septal defects in infants. J Thorac Cardiovasc Surg 75:346, 1978.
30. Milo S, Yen Ho S, Wilkinson JL, Anderson RH: Surgical anatomy and atrioventricular conduction tissues of hearts with isolated ventricular septal defects. J Thorac Cardiovasc Surg 79:244, 1980.
31. Mitchell SC, Korones SB, Berendes HW: Congenital heart disease in 56,109 births. Incidence and natural history. Circulation 43:323, 1971.
32. Muller WH Jr, Damman JF Jr: The treatment of certain congenital malformations of the heart by creation of pulmonic stenosis to reduce pulmonary hypertension and pulmonary flow. Surg Gynecol Obstet 95:312, 1952.
33. Murphy DA, Poirier N: A technique of aortic valvuloplasty for aortic insufficiency associated with ventricular septal defect. J Thorac Cardiovasc Surg 64:800, 1972.
34. Nadas AS, Blount SG Jr: Management of ventricular septal defects in adults. Chest 74:3, 1978.
35. Nadas AS, Thilenius OG, LaFarge CG, Hauck AJ: Ventricular septal defect with aortic regurgitation. Medical and pathologic aspects. Circulation 29:862, 1964.
36. Rein JG, Freed MD, Norwood WI, Castaneda AR: Early and late results of closure of ventricular septal defect in infancy. Ann Thorac Surg 24:19, 1977.

37. Sanfelippo PM, DuShane JW, McGoon DC, Danielson GK: Ventricular septal defect and aortic insufficiency. Ann Thorac Surg 17:213, 1974.
38. Sealy WC, Hackel DB, Seaber AV: A study of methods for interruption of the His bundle. J Thorac Cardiovasc Surg 73:424, 1977.
39. Serwer GA, Armstrong BE, Anderson PAW, Sherman D, Benson DW Jr, Edwards SB: Use of contrast echocardiography for evaluation of right ventricular hemodynamics in the presence of ventricular septal defects. Circulation 58:327, 1978.
40. Seybold-Epting W, Reul GJ Jr, Hallman GL, Cooley DA: Repair of ventricular septal defect after pulmonary artery banding. J Thorac Cardiovasc Surg 71:392, 1976.
41. Singh AK, deLeval MR, Stark J: Left ventriculotomy for closure of muscular ventricular septal defects: treatment of choice. Ann Surg 186:577, 1977.
42. Somerville J, Brandao A, Ross DN: Aortic regurgitation with ventricular septal defect. Surgical management and clinical features. Circulation 41:317, 1970.
43. Spencer FC, Doyle EF, Danilowicz DA, Bahnson HT, Weldon CS: Long-term evaluation of aortic valvuloplasty for aortic insufficiency and ventricular septal defect. J Thorac Cardiovasc Surg 65:15, 1973.
44. Starr A, Menashe V, Dotter C: Successful correction of aortic insufficiency associated with ventricular septal defect. Surg Gynecol Obstet 111:71, 1960.
45. Stirling GR, Stanley PH, Lillehei CW: The effects of cardiac bypass and ventriculotomy upon right ventricular function. Surg Forum 8:433, 1957.
46. Suzuki Y, Ishizawa E, Tanaka S, Itoh T, Satoh K, Koizumi S, Tadokoro M, Horiuchi T, Satoh T, Kanoh I: Surgical treatment of large ventricular septal defect with pulmonary hypertension in the first 24 months of life. Ann Thorac Surg 22:228, 1976.
47. Tandler J: Anatomie des Herzens, Jena, Gustav Fischer, 1913, p 64.
48. Tatsuno K, Konno S, Ando M, Sakakibara S: Pathogenetic mechanisms of prolapsing aortic valve and aortic regurgitation associated with ventricular septal defect. Anatomical, angiographic and surgical considerations. Circulation 48:1028, 1973.
49. Titus JL: Normal anatomy of the human cardiac conduction system. Mayo Clin Proc. 48:24, 1973.
50. Titus JL, Daugherty GW, Edwards JE: Anatomy of the atrioventricular conduction system in ventricular septal defect. Circulation 28:72, 1963.
51. Truex RC, Bishof JK: Conduction system in human hearts with interventricular septal defects. J Thorac Surg 35:421, 1958.
52. Truex RC, Smythe MQ: Reconstruction of the human atrioventricular node. Anat Rec 158:11, 1964.
53. Trusler GA, Moes CAF, Kidd BSL: Repair of ventricular septal defect with aortic insufficiency. J Thorac Cardiovasc Surg 66:394, 1973.
54. Trusler GA, Mustard WT: A method of banding the pulmonary artery for large isolated ventricular septal defect with and without transposition of the great arteries. Ann Thorac Surg 13:351, 1972.
55. Utley JR: Hemodynamic observations during and after pulmonary artery banding. Ann Thorac Surg 15:493, 1973.
56. Van Praagh R, McNamara JJ: Anatomic types of ventricular septal defect with aortic insufficiency: diagnostic and surgical considerations. Am Heart J 75:604, 1968.
57. Wenink ACG, Oppenheimer-Dekker A, Moulaert AJ: Muscular ventricular septal defects: a reappraisal of the anatomy. Am J Cardiol 43:259, 1979.

22 Tetralogy of Fallot

It is now a quarter century since total correction of tetralogy of Fallot was first reported by Lillehei[41] and demonstrated to be a feasible, low-risk operation by Kirklin.[33] During that time significant advances have occurred. Such advances, however, have not completely resolved the continuing controversy over when surgical intervention is indicated and what surgical approach should be taken—the two-stage approach of a palliative procedure to increase pulmonary blood flow followed by later total correction or the one-stage approach of primary total correction. Whatever approach is taken, surgery has an extremely important role in tetralogy of Fallot. The life expectancy without surgery is extremely poor: one-third of patients will die before 1 year, half before 3 years, and only one-quarter will live to 10 years.[6]

Indications

Initial Palliation Versus Primary Total Correction

Alfred Blalock,[9] in his discussion of Lillehei's paper in 1955, correctly predicted that "the mortality accompanying the anastomotic procedure in the treatment of tetralogy of Fallot will remain lower for quite some time than that accompanying the direct attack under vision." Such was the case for many years in many institutions. As recently as 1972 it was the policy of Puga, DuShane, and McGoon,[52] of the Mayo Clinic, "to defer open correction until the child is 5 to 10 years old, using surgical palliation when necessary for the younger child who presents with severe symptoms."

However, an increasing number of reports[1,4,14,18,49,53,58,64] appearing during the early 1970s documented the fact that primary total correction of tetralogy of Fallot during infancy could be performed in properly selected patients with a mortality below 10% and with excellent late results. At the same time, refinement of the Blalock-Taussig operation (Chapter 13) made it a safe and effective procedure in the infant,[3,60] continuing the controversy over the proper surgical approach. In addition, nonoperative therapy with propranolol has been described,[23,27] although it is least applicable to the infant with fixed stenosis at the pulmonary anulus.[16] Propranolol is not used at our institution for treatment of tetralogy of Fallot.

Proper timing of surgical intervention and proper choice of surgical procedure in tetralogy of Fallot are based on an understanding of the spectrum of anatomy and physiology that can occur.[10] The anatomic variability in tetralogy of Fallot occurs in the pulmonary outflow tract and pulmonary arteries: the anatomy that does not cause symptoms until childhood usually consists of infundibular stenosis with mild or no stenosis at the pulmonary anulus, main pulmonary arteries, or branch pulmonary arteries; the anatomy that causes symptoms and severe hypoxemia during infancy usually consists of stenosis at the pulmonary anulus[14] and frequently is associated with some hypoplasia of the main pulmonary artery as well. Hypoplasia of the branch pulmonary arteries may also be present. Infundibular stenosis often is mild in this latter subset of tetralogy of Fallot.[58]

Although small size,[31] young age, and severity of hypoxemia may correlate with increased risk of primary total correction, the most significant variable appears to be the degree of hypoplasia of the main and branch pulmonary arteries and therefore the capacitance of the pulmonary artery system. A poorly developed pulmonary artery system will not accommodate the total cardiac output resulting from closure of the VSD. This causes right ventricular failure and death from low cardiac output. Therefore, it has been our objective for years to identify those patients with underdeveloped pulmonary artery systems and to perform initial palliation in this group in infancy.[58] Patients who have an adequate main pulmonary artery and adequate branch pulmonary arteries undergo total correction at the onset of cyanosis or hypoxic spells.

A number of methods have been described to define those patients with a hypoplastic pulmonary arterial system. We and others have used the ratio of the main pulmonary artery to the ascending aorta and perform a palliative operation if the ratio is less than 0.3. Blackstone, Kirklin and colleagues[7] have described a formula using the ratio of the right and left pulmonary arteries to the descending thoracic aorta. Tucker, Ebert, and co-workers[62] use the ratio of the right pulmonary artery to the ascending aorta, choosing initial palliation if the ratio is less than 0.3.

In the presence of adequate pulmonary arteries our only general contraindication to total correction of tetralogy of Fallot in the infant is an anomalous anterior descending coronary artery arising from the right coronary artery. However, others[63] do not consider this a contraindication.

The symptomatic patient with tetralogy of Fallot therefore undergoes total correction regardless of size or age if the main pulmonary artery/ascending aorta ratio is over 0.3 and if the origin of the anterior descending is normal. This encompasses the majority of patients. The remaining patients undergo a palliative procedure.

Reoperation

Reoperation is indicated if a hemodynamically significant ventricular septal defect is present ($Q_p/Q_s > 2:1$),[54] a large right ventricular outflow gradient persists (over 60 mm Hg), or there is an aneurysm of the right ventricular outflow patch. An aneurysm of the outflow patch is usually associated with an outflow gradient. Reoperation for residual lesions after tetralogy repair can be performed with the same low mortality and morbidity associated with the original operation,[15] if serious deterioration of right ventricular function has not occurred. Periodic follow-up of all patients postoperatively and early performance of studies if hemodynamic abnormality is suspected will prevent neglected situations.

Surgical Strategy

Choice of Palliative Procedure
We have detailed the reasoning underlying our choice of systemic-pulmonary shunts in Chapter 13. It is our recent practice to perform more Blalock-Taussig shunts, although we continue to perform Waterston shunts on occasion. There is growing evidence that a properly performed Blalock-Taussig[22] or Waterston[2] shunt results in growth of the pulmonary arteries and that subsequent correction can be performed at low risk.[18]

Tetralogy of Fallot offers an additional method of increasing pulmonary blood flow: patching across the pulmonary anulus, either leaving the VSD open[63] or partially closing it with a perforated patch.[47] This approach can result in symmetric growth of the pulmonary arteries.[26,63] More time will be necessary to determine how this method of palliation compares with the classic procedures, but it is unlikely to supplant the shunt operations.

Closure of Systemic-Pulmonary Shunts
The patency of shunts should be confirmed at catheterization. A continuous murmur may be due to bronchial collaterals and does not invariably indicate the presence of a patent shunt. The right-sided Blalock-Taussig shunt is usually easy to close at the time of total correction. The approach is intrapericardial.[34] The subclavian artery is located just above its junction with the right main pulmonary artery; this is usually medial to the superior vena cava. The superior vena cava is dissected, encircled, and retracted laterally. The aorta is retracted medially. An incision is made in the posterior pericardium over the palpated subclavian artery, and the artery is dissected and encircled; it is tied after cardiopulmonary bypass is begun.

Dissection and encirclement of the left-sided Blalock-Taussig shunt are more formidable. The approach is outside the pericardium over the left pulmonary artery, with dissection guided by the palpable thrill.[34]

Closure of a properly constructed Waterston shunt can usually be accomplished through the ascending aorta. If the right pulmonary artery is kinked or narrowed, it should be detached from the aorta and patched with pericardium if necessary.[25]

Our preferred technique for closure of a Potts anastomosis involves hypothermic perfusion and circulatory arrest with closure through the left pulmonary artery.[32] The artery is opened directly opposite the shunt.

Myocardial Preservation
Cold crystalloid cardioplegic arrest is our method of myocardial preservation (Chapter 6). This technique creates a flaccid myocardium, markedly facilitating the exposure of the ventricular septal defect.

Decision Regarding Transanular Patch
Relief of resistance to right ventricular emptying is an essential component of successful repair. It is desirable, if possible, to achieve this without producing pulmonary insufficiency. However, the relief of outflow obstruction is more important than avoidance of pulmonary insufficiency; for this reason there has been continuing evaluation of methods that can predict the necessity of a transanular patch.

Empirical estimates at the time of repair and measuring the ratio of right ventricular to left ventricular pressure while temporarily discontinuing cardiopulmonary bypass following repair have both been used. However, a more scientific and predictable method of determining the necessity of a transanular patch during the initial repair is desirable. Such a method has been described by Pacifico, Kirklin, and Blackstone,[50] basing the decision for primary enlargement of the pulmonary valve ring on a weight-related or surface area-related "minimum pulmonary valve ring diameter." This method is based on the studies of normal pulmonary anulus circumference by Rowlatt, Rimoldi, and Lev[56] and is a predictable method.[8]

At operation we pass calibrated dilators through the pulmonary valve from below and generally seek a normal anulus diameter, using the weight-related chart of Pacifico and colleagues,[50] patching across the anulus whenever indicated. We keep the chart posted in our operating room and find it useful for assessing all forms of pulmonary stenosis as well as determining the size of the patch. If there is any question, we are liberal in our use of a patch, since it appears that a transanular patch has little if any effect on early or late results.[30,43]

Associated Anomalies

Patent Ductus Arteriosus
This is ligated at the time of open repair as described in Chapter 11.

Anomalous Coronary Artery
The anterior descending artery arises from the right coronary artery in approximately 5% of patients with tetralogy of Fallot,[17] crossing the right ventricular outflow tract in a position where it can be transected by a vertical ventriculotomy. Such transection frequently results in myocardial infarction and death. As noted earlier, we consider an anomalous anterior descending artery a contraindication to repair in infancy.

Injury to an anomalous anterior descending can be avoided by repair through the right atrium[19] or by performing a transverse ventriculotomy caudal to the artery.[51] If the outflow tract cannot be adequately enlarged through such a ventriculotomy, a conduit can be placed over the anomalous artery to the pulmonary artery.[44]

Atrial Septal Defect or Patent Foramen Ovale
Atrial septal communications should be searched for, either through the tricuspid valve via the ventriculotomy or through an atriotomy, and closed if present.

Single Pulmonary Artery
This condition can be congenital or can be caused by a systemic-pulmonary shunt. Successful repair is possible. Some recommend a valved conduit as a standard component of the repair.[46]

Absent Pulmonary Valve
This condition is usually associated with dilation of the pulmonary arteries and tracheobronchial obstruction. Pulmonary difficulties are often more serious than the intracardiac pathophysiology.[37,45] Repair involving insertion of a tube graft between the main pulmonary artery and distal pulmonary arteries has been recommended,[42] although often this is not necessary.[57] Our practice has been to treat tetralogy with absent pulmonary valve the same as the more common forms of tetralogy.

Complete Atrioventricular Canal
This lesion can be corrected, when it occurs in association with tetralogy of Fallot, by a combined approach through the atrium and ventricle.[67]

Surgical Anatomy

Fallot[20,21] described the tetralogy in 1888: ventricular septal defect, infundibular pulmonic stenosis, dextroposition of the aorta, right ventricular hypertrophy. There is a variation in the anatomy of tetralogy of Fallot, which can cause controversy over the proper classification of some anatomic subsets. For most cases, however, there is little question over proper classification.

The anatomic defects as described by Fallot invariably result in equal ventricular pressures. Right-to-left shunting at the ventricular level usually occurs and may be constant or intermittent.

Ventricular Septal Defect

The ventricular septal defect is large, usually the diameter of the ascending aorta or larger. It is subaortic in location, in the anterior portion of the muscular septum, anterior to the pars membranacea (Fig. 22-1). It is below the posterior part of the right coronary cusp and the anterior part of the noncoronary cusp.[40]

The ventricular septal defect, as viewed by the surgeon through an infundibular incision, is bordered anteriorly, inferiorly, and superiorly by septal musculature. The posterior border is often formed by tissue at the base of the septal leaflet of the tricuspid valve, and may also contain some of the pars membranacea as well as a portion of the aortic anulus. The superior border is the crista supraventricularis, also referred to as conus septum.

Conduction System

Lev's careful studies[38,39] of the architecture of the conduction system in congenital heart disease, particularly tetralogy of Fallot, have greatly contributed to our knowledge. He has shown that, in tetralogy of Fallot, the AV bundle

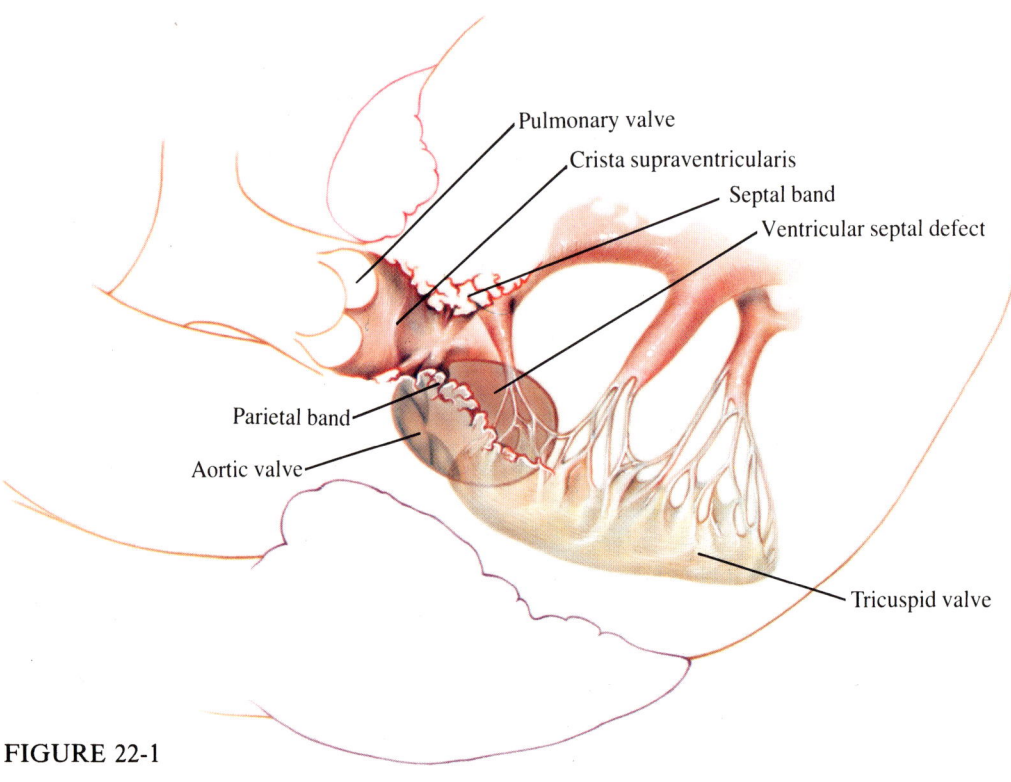

FIGURE 22-1

penetrates the central fibrous body as the conus musculature inserts on the central fibrous body. If there is an upward extension of the central fibrous body (pars membranacea), then the bundle may lie at the base of this portion of the ventricular septum. The bundle lays on the left side of the septum as it reaches the level of the ventricular septal defect. Here it is flattened and widened out, lying on the left side of the septum below the defect.

The left-sided location of the bundle makes it possible to place sutures in the crest of the inferior border of the ventricular septal defect without producing heart block.

Right Ventricular Outflow Obstruction

A variable amount of pulmonic stenosis is always present at the infundibular level. Approximately one-third of cases will have stenosis only at the infundibulum.[29] The next most frequent location of pulmonic stenosis is at the valvar or anular level. The pulmonic valve is often bicuspid. Stenosis at the level of the main pulmonary artery or the branch pulmonary arteries may also occur.

Technique

A vertical incision is made in the infundibulum (Fig. 22-2). We prefer a vertical incision because it exposes the infundibular stenosis and the VSD well and, in contrast to a transverse incision, can easily be extended across the pulmonary anulus if necessary.

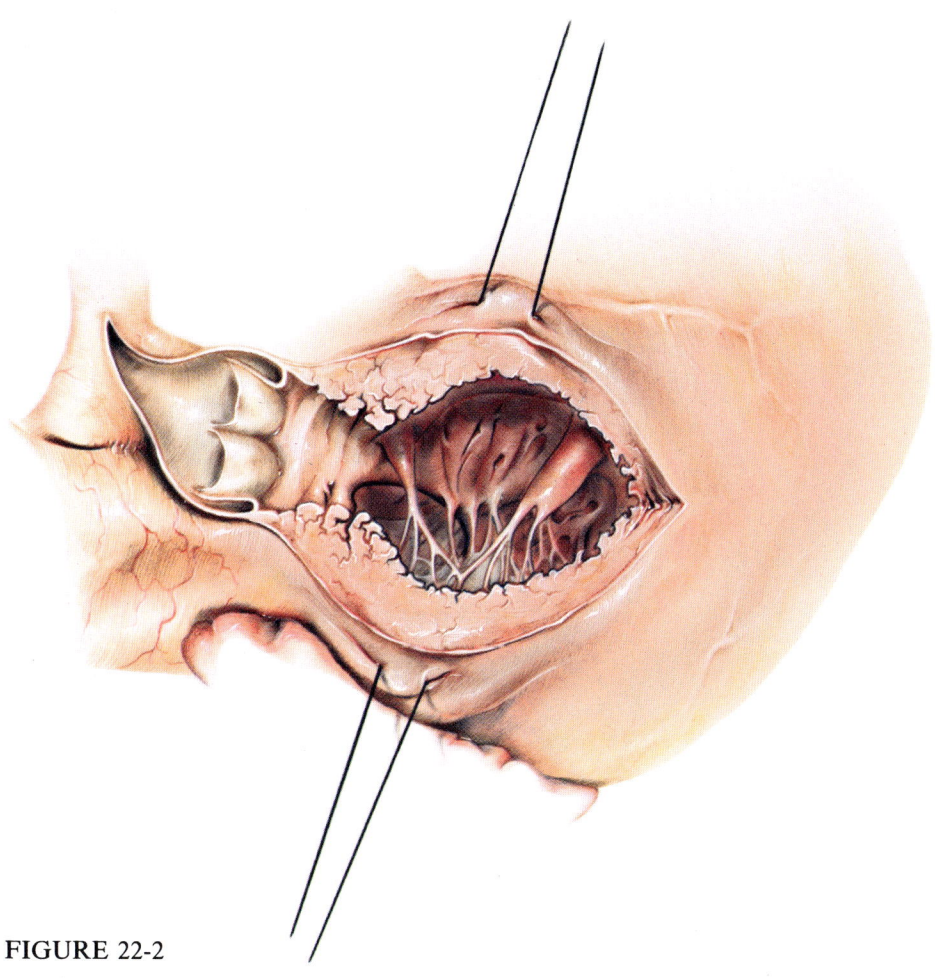

FIGURE 22-2

Tetralogy of Fallot

The constricting septal bands (Fig. 22-3) and parietal bands (Fig. 22-4) are incised and excised (Fig. 22-5). The bands are frequently tightly packed, but a right-angle clamp can be insinuated behind them, aiding incision and excision.

None of the crista supraventricularis (conus septum) is excised; such excision can injure the underlying aortic valve and also jeopardizes secure anchoring of sutures around the superior border of the VSD patch.

The pulmonary valve and anulus are inspected from below, and Bakes or Hegar dilators are passed to calibrate the valve and anulus diameter,[50] as discussed earlier in this chapter. If the pulmonary anulus and pulmonary artery are of good size but there is valvular stenosis, a pulmonic commissurotomy is performed through a separate pulmonary arteriotomy. In the presence of a small anulus and pulmonary artery, the ventriculotomy is extended across the anulus onto the pulmonary artery as far as necessary, frequently into the left main branch.

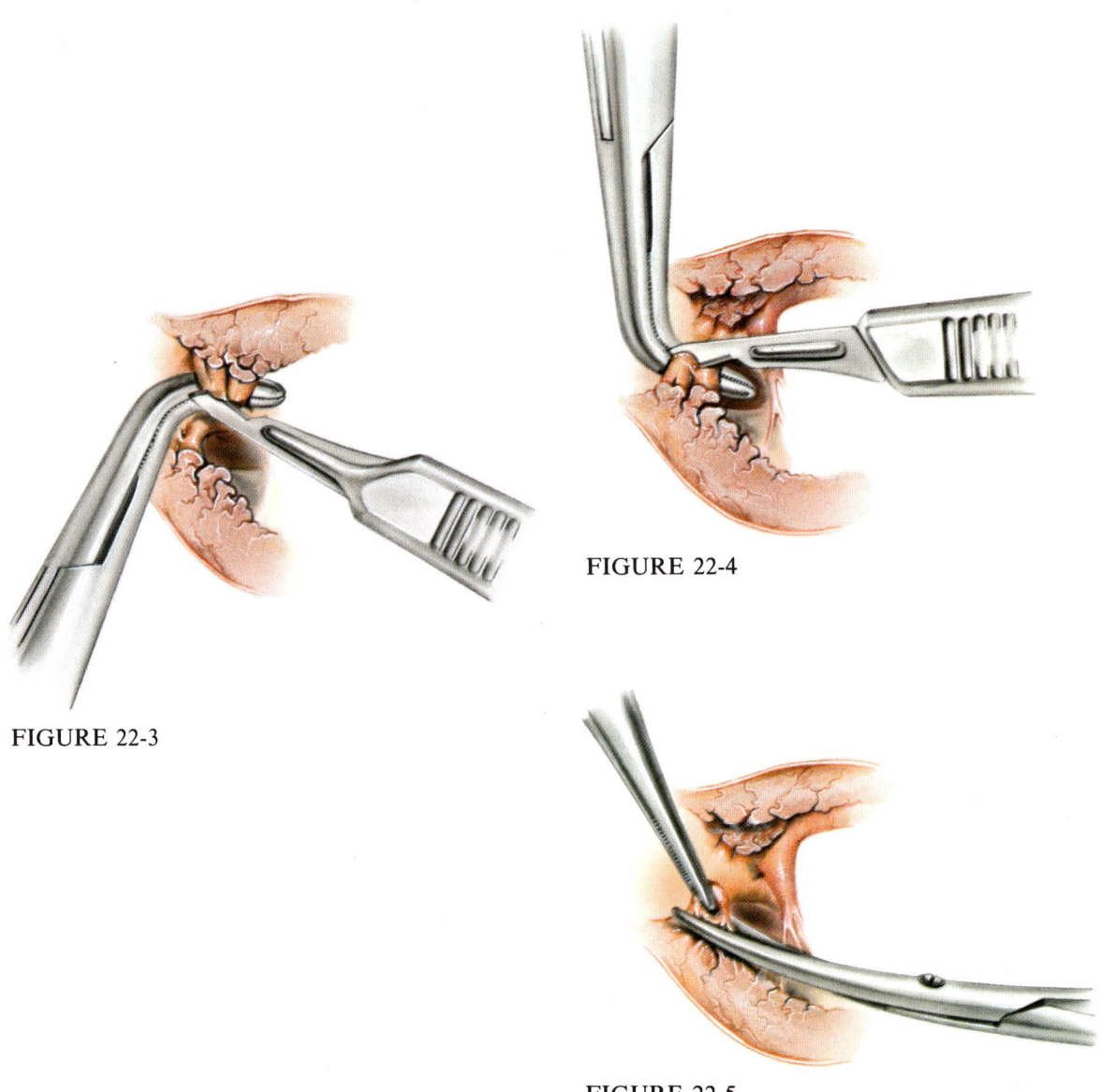

FIGURE 22-3

FIGURE 22-4

FIGURE 22-5

Incision and excision of the septal and parietal bands help expose the ventricular septal defect. Exposure is further aided by placing a small intracardiac sucker through the defect, with retraction to the left (Fig. 22-6).

Closure of the ventricular septal defect is with a patch of Teflon or knitted Dacron double-velour, using interrupted 4-0 silk sutures on small half-circle needles.

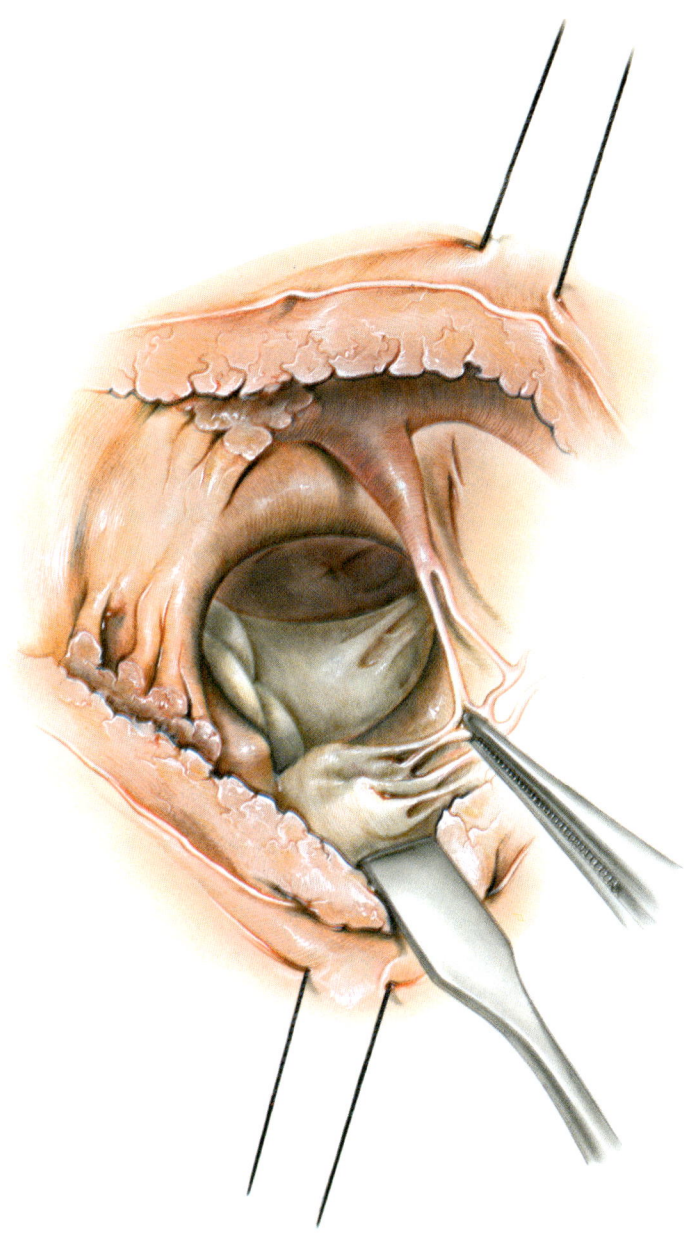

FIGURE 22-6

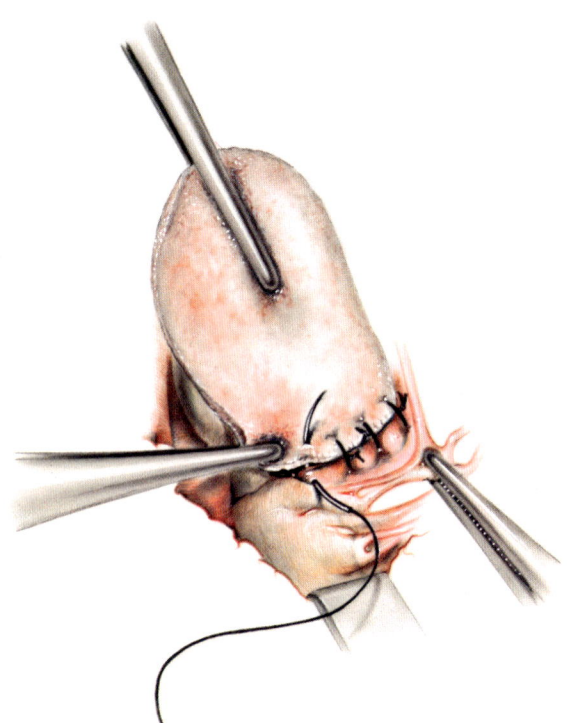

FIGURE 22-7

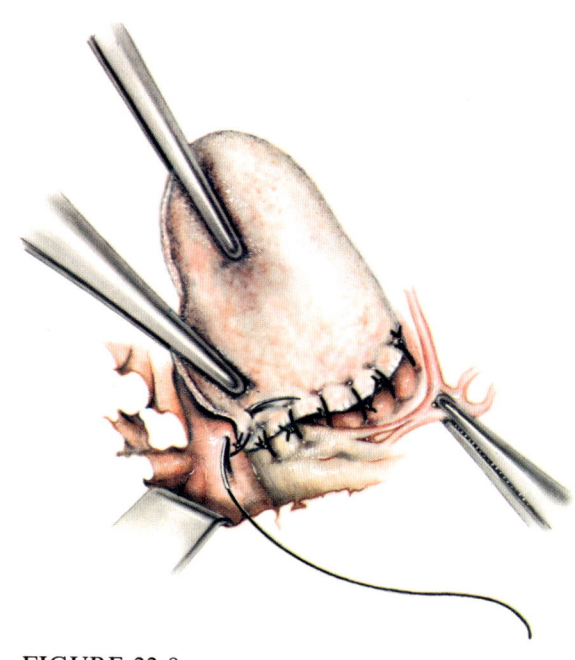

FIGURE 22-8

The first suture is placed in the midportion of the caudal rim of the defect (Fig. 22-7). Forceps never grasp the defect margin. The patch, slightly larger in diameter than the aortic root, is tied into place.

Sutures are placed in a clockwise direction, into the tricuspid anulus (Fig. 22-8) and the aortic anulus if extreme overriding is present. No attempt is made to stay away from the defect margin. Sutures are placed in the parietal limb of the crista supraventricularis (Fig. 22-9).

Closure then begins again at the first suture and moves counterclockwise up to the crista, with deep sutures in the muscular margin (Fig. 22-10). Sutures are then placed attaching the patch to the crista (Fig. 22-11).

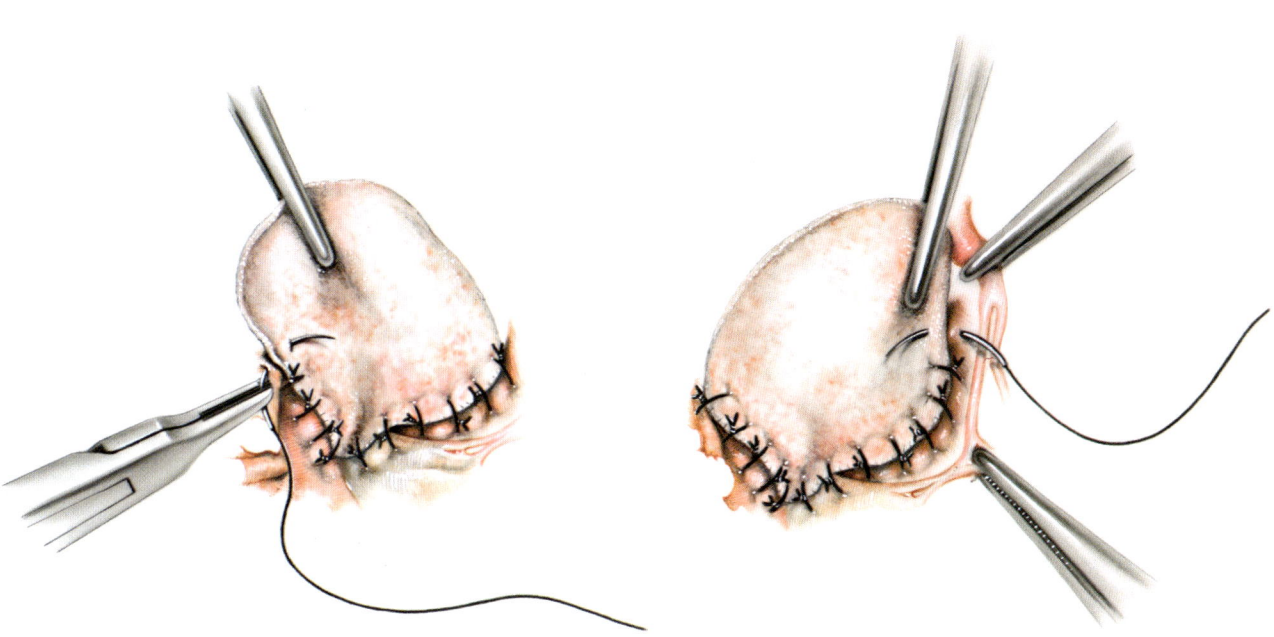

FIGURE 22-9

FIGURE 22-10

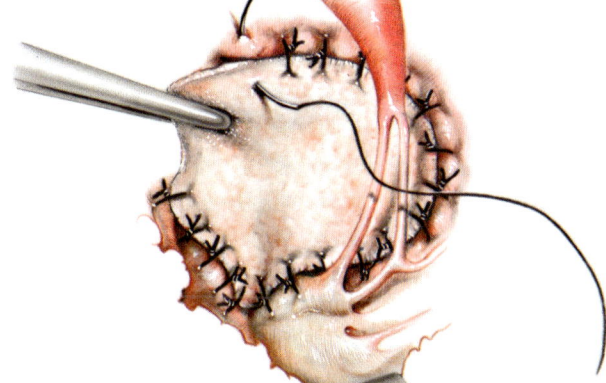

FIGURE 22-11

If the pulmonary valve diameter is adequate, the infundibular outflow area is assessed. If the ventricular edges cannot be approximated easily over a Hegar dilator the size of the patient's pulmonary valve orifice, a patch, usually of pericardium in infants, is placed over the infundibulum. If transanular patching is necessary, it is frequently begun on or at the base of the left pulmonary artery and carried across the anulus onto the ventricle (Fig. 22-12).

Prior to decannulation, pressures are measured in the right ventricle. An acceptable right ventricular–systemic artery pressure ratio is 0.75 or less.

Late Results

Clinical Status

Late survival at five to ten years following correction of tetralogy of Fallot is 95%.[13,35,51] The vast majority of patients are asymptomatic. Sunderland and co-workers,[61] in a study from our institution of 27 survivors of correction in infancy, found all to be asymptomatic. Similarly excellent results have been reported by others.[35,51] Garson and colleagues[24] have shown that over 80% of adults who undergo correction during childhood can lead a normal life without impairment of intellect, exercise tolerance, or fertility.

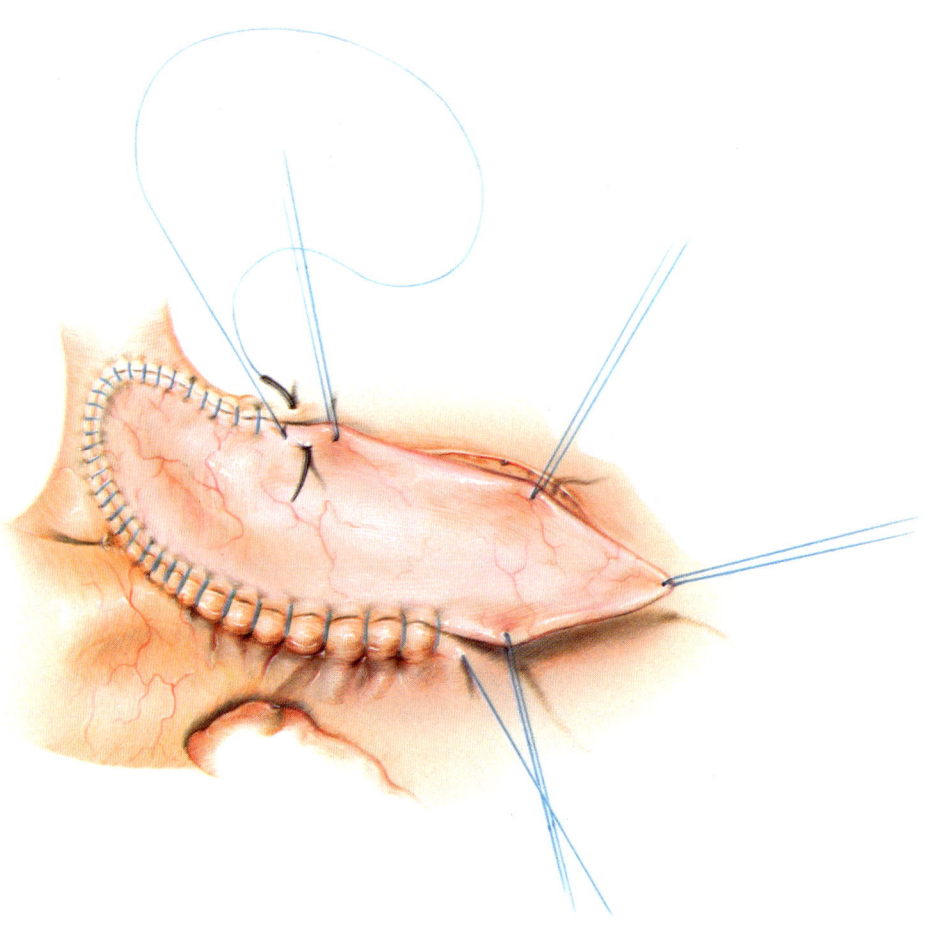

FIGURE 22-12

Hemodynamic Status

Most patients have minor hemodynamic abnormalities after correction. They still are able, however, to have normal or nearly normal cardiovascular responses to maximal exercise as measured by cardiac output, maximal oxygen consumption, and left ventricular ejection fraction.[55] The most common hemodynamic abnormalities are mild right ventricular hypertension (30–45 mm Hg), a small gradient between the right ventricle and pulmonary artery (10–20 mm Hg), and pulmonary regurgitation.[11,12,61] Bristow and colleagues[11] have demonstrated a stable hemodynamic status in patients for up to ten years.

Electrophysiologic Changes

Minor electrophysiologic changes are the rule after repair of tetralogy of Fallot. More severe changes are much less frequent but are an area of controversy, both regarding their significance and their proper management.

Right bundle branch block (RBBB) occurs in 85%–95% of patients after repair of tetralogy of Fallot.[28,59] As an isolated electrophysiologic change it is entirely benign.

Right bundle branch block with left anterior hemiblock (RBBB+LAH) occurs much less frequently, in 8%–18%.[28,59,66] There are conflicting reports regarding the prognosis of RBBB+LAH. Wolff and co-workers[65] reported sudden death in 12.5% of patients with RBBB+LAH and in 2% of patients without the pattern. However, Gillette[28] and Steeg[59] report two separate series of patients with RBBB+LAH without any late deaths. The different prognoses may be due to different sites of conduction injury.[36]

Gillette and colleagues[28] report premature ventricular contractions (PVCs) to be associated with sudden death. In addition, all of the patients who died had significant congestive heart failure. They recommend treating postoperative patients who have PVCs with quinidine or propranolol.

There is not enough information available at this time to make sound recommendations as to whether patients, other than those with complete heart block, should have prophylactic or therapeutic pacing.

References

1. Adams P, Radley-Smith R, Yacoub M: Primary total correction of Fallot's tetralogy below the age of 2 years. Br Heart J 36:1036, 1974.
2. Alfieri O, Locatelli G, Bianchi T, Vanini V, Parenzan L: Repair of tetralogy of Fallot after Waterston anastomosis. J Thorac Cardiovasc Surg 77:826, 1979.
3. Arciniegas E, Farooki ZQ, Hakimi M, Green EW: Results of two-stage surgical treatment of tetralogy of Fallot. J Thorac Cardiovasc Surg 79:876, 1980.
4. Barratt-Boyes BG, Neutze JM: Primary repair of tetralogy of Fallot in infancy using profound hypothermia with circulatory arrest and limited cardiopulmonary bypass: a comparison with conventional two stage management. Ann Surg 178:406, 1973.
5. Berry BE, McGoon DC: Total correction for tetralogy of Fallot with anomalous coronary artery. Surgery 74:894, 1973.
6. Bertranou EG, Blackstone EH, Hazelrig JB, Turner ME Jr, Kirklin JW: Life expectancy without surgery in tetralogy of Fallot. Am J Cardiol 41:458, 1978.
7. Blackstone EH, Kirklin JW, Bertranou EG, Labrosse CJ, Soto B, Bargeron LM: Preoperative prediction from cineangiograms of post-repair right ventricular pressure in tetralogy of Fallot. J Thorac Cardiovasc Surg 78:542, 1979.
8. Blackstone EH, Kirklin JW, Pacifico AD: Decision-making in repair of tetralogy of Fallot based on intraoperative measurements of pulmonary arterial outflow tract. J Thorac Cardiovasc Surg 77:526, 1979.
9. Blalock A: Discussion of Lillehei et al: Direct vision intracardiac surgical correc-

tion of the tetralogy of Fallot, pentalogy of Fallot and pulmonary atresia defects. Ann Surg 142:418, 1955.
10. Bonchek LI, Starr A, Sunderland CO, Menashe VD: Natural history of tetralogy of Fallot in infancy: clinical classification and therapeutic implications. Circulation 48:392, 1973.
11. Bristow JD, Kloster FE, Lees MH, Menashe VD, Griswold HE, Starr A: Serial cardiac catheterizations and exercise hemodynamics after correction of tetralogy of Fallot. Average follow-up 13 months and 7 years after operation. Circulation 41:1057, 1970.
12. Burnell RH, Woodson RD, Lees MH, Bristow JD, Starr A: Results of correction of tetralogy of Fallot in children under four years of age. J Thorac Cardiovasc Surg 57:153, 1969.
13. Calder AL, Barratt-Boyes BG, Brandt PWT, Neutze JM: Postoperative evaluation of patients with tetralogy of Fallot repaired in infancy. Including criteria for use of outflow patching and radiologic assessment of pulmonary regurgitation. J Thorac Cardiovasc Surg 77:704, 1979.
14. Castaneda AR, Freed MD, Williams RG, Norwood WI: Repair of tetralogy of Fallot in infancy. J Thorac Cardiovasc Surg 74:372, 1977.
15. Castaneda AR, Sade RM, Lamberti J, Nicoloff DM: Reoperation for residual defects after repair of tetralogy of Fallot. Surgery 76:1010, 1974.
16. Cumming GR: Propranolol in tetralogy of Fallot. Editorial. Circulation 41:13, 1970.
17. Dabizzi RP, Caprioli G, Aiazzi L, Castelli C, Baldrighi G, Parenzan L, Baldrighi V: Distribution and anomalies of coronary arteries in tetralogy of Fallot. Circulation 61:95, 1980.
18. Daily PO, Stinson EB, Griepp RB, Shumway NE: Tetralogy of Fallot: choice of surgical procedure. J Thorac Cardiovasc Surg 75:338, 1978.
19. Edmunds LH Jr, Saxena NC, Friedman S, Rashkind JW, Dodd PF: Transatrial repair of tetralogy of Fallot. Surgery 80:681, 1976.
20. Fallot A: Contribution of l'anatomie pathologique de la maladie bleue (cyanose cardiaque). Marseille Med 25:77, 138, 207, 270, 341, 403, 1888.
21. Fallot A: Contribution to the pathologic anatomy of morbus caeruleus (translated summary). *In* Willins, Keys (eds): Cardiac Classics. St Louis, CV Mosby Co, 1941, pp 689, 690.
22. Gale AW, Arciniegas E, Green EW, Blackstone EH, Kirklin JW: Growth of the pulmonary anulus and pulmonary arteries after the Blalock-Taussig shunt. J Thorac Cardiovasc Surg 77:459, 1979.
23. Garson A Jr, Gorry GA, McNamara DG, Cooley DA: The surgical decision in tetralogy of Fallot: weighing risks and benefits with decision analysis. Am J Cardiol 45:108, 1980.
24. Garson A, Nihill MR, McNamara DG, Cooley DA: Status of the adult and adolescent after repair of tetralogy of Fallot. Circulation 59:1232, 1979.
25. Gay WA Jr, Ebert PA: Aorta-to-right pulmonary artery anastomosis causing obstruction of the right pulmonary artery: management during correction of tetralogy of Fallot. Ann Thorac Surg 16:402, 1973.
26. Gill GC, Moodie DS, McGoon DC: Staged surgical management of pulmonary atresia with diminutive pulmonary arteries. J Thorac Cardiovasc Surg 73:436, 1977.
27. Gillette PC, Garson A, Eterovic E, Nehces W, Mullins CE, McNamara DG: Results of oral propranolol in infants and children. J Pediatr 86:170, 1978.
28. Gillette PC, Yeoman MA, Mullins CE, McNamara DG: Sudden death after repair of tetralogy of Fallot: electrocardiographic and electrophysiologic abnormalities. Circulation 56:566, 1977.
29. Howe A, Rastelli GC, Ritter DG, DuShane JW, McGoon DC: Management of the right ventricular outflow tract in severe tetralogy of Fallot. J Thorac Cardiovasc Surg 60:131, 1970.
30. Jones EL, Conti CR, Neill CA, Gott VL, Brawley RK, Haller JA: Long-term evaluation of tetralogy patients with pulmonary valvular insufficiency resulting

from outflow-patch correction across the pulmonic annulus. Circulation 48(Suppl III):III-11, 1973.
31. Kirklin JW, Blackstone EH, Pacifico AD, Brown RN, Bargeron LM: Routine primary repair vs two-stage repair of tetralogy of Fallot. Circulation 60:373, 1979.
32. Kirklin JW, Devloo RA: Hypothermic perfusion and circulatory arrest for surgical correction of tetralogy of Fallot with previously constructed Potts' anastomosis. Dis Chest 39:87, 1961.
33. Kirklin JW, Ellis FH, McGoon DC, DuShane JW, Swan JC: Surgical treatment for the tetralogy of Fallot by open intracardiac repair. J Thorac Cardiovasc Surg 37:22, 1959.
34. Kirklin JW, Payne WS: Surgical treatment for tetralogy of Fallot after previous anastomosis of systemic to pulmonary artery. Surg Gynecol Obstet 110:707, 1960.
35. Kirklin JW, Wallace RB, McGoon DC, DuShane JW: Early and late results after intracardiac repair of tetralogy of Fallot. Ann Surg 162:578, 1965.
36. Krongard E: Prognosis for patients with congenital heart disease and postoperative intraventricular conduction defects. Circulation 57:867, 1978.
37. Lakier JB, Stanger P, Heymann MA, Hoffman JIE, Rudolph AM: Tetralogy of Fallot with absent pulmonary valve. Natural history and hemodynamic considerations. Circulation 50:167, 1974.
38. Lev M: The architecture of the conduction system in congenital heart disease. II. Tetralogy of Fallot. Arch Pathol Lab Med 67:572, 1959.
39. Lev M: Conduction system in congenital heart disease. Am J Cardiol 21:619, 1968.
40. Lev M, Eckner RAO: The pathologic anatomy of tetralogy of Fallot and its variations. Dis Chest 45:251, 1964.
41. Lillehei CW, Cohen M, Warden HE, Reed RC, Aust JB, Dewall RA, Varco RL: Direct vision intracardiac surgical correction of the tetralogy of Fallot, pentalogy of Fallot and pulmonary atresia defects. Ann Surg 142:418, 1955.
42. Litwin SB, Rosenthal A, Fellows K: Surgical management of young infants with tetralogy of Fallot, absence of the pulmonary valve, and respiratory distress. J Thorac Cardiovasc Surg 65:552, 1973.
43. McGoon DC: Discussion of Pacifico et al: Surgical management of pulmonary stenosis in tetralogy of Fallot. J Thorac Cardiovasc Surg 74:382, 1977.
44. Meyer J, Chiarello L, Hallman GL, Cooley DA: Coronary artery anomalies in patients with tetralogy of Fallot. J Thorac Cardiovasc Surg 69:373, 1975.
45. Miller RA, Lev M, Paul MH: Congenital absence of the pulmonary valve: the clinical syndrome of tetralogy of Fallot with pulmonary regurgitation. Circulation 26:266, 1962.
46. Mistrot JJ, Bernhard WF, Rosenthal A, Castaneda AR: Tetralogy of Fallot with a single pulmonary artery: operative repair. Ann Thorac Surg 23:249, 1977.
47. Norwood WI, Rosenthal A, Castaneda AR: Tetralogy of Fallot with acquired pulmonary atresia and hypoplasia of pulmonary arteries. J Thorac Cardiovasc Surg 72:454, 1976.
48. Oku H, Shirotani H, Yokoyama T, Tokota Y, Kawai J, Mori A, Kanzaki Y, Makino S, Ando F, Setsuie N: Postoperative size of the right ventricular outflow tract and optimal age in complete repair of tetralogy of Fallot. Ann Thorac Surg 25:322, 1978.
49. Pacifico AD, Bargeron LM, Kirklin JW: Primary total correction of tetralogy of Fallot in children less than four years of age. Circulation 48:1085, 1973.
50. Pacifico AD, Kirklin JW, Blackstone EH: Surgical management of pulmonary stenosis in tetralogy of Fallot. J Thorac Cardiovasc Surg 74:382, 1977.
51. Poirer RA, McGoon DC, Danielson GK, Wallace RB, Ritter DG, Moodie DS, Wiltse CG: Late results after repair of tetralogy of Fallot. J Thorac Cardiovasc Surg 73:900, 1977.
52. Puga FJ, DuShane JW, McGoon DC: Treatment of tetralogy of Fallot in children less than 4 years of age. J Thorac Cardiovasc Surg 64:247, 1972.
53. Rees GM, Starr A: Total correction of Fallot's tetralogy in patients aged less than 1 year. Br Heart J 35:898, 1973.

54. Rocchini AP, Rosenthal A, Freed M, Castaneda AR, Nadas AS: Chronic congestive heart failure after repair of tetralogy of Fallot. Circulation 56:305, 1977.
55. Rosing DR, Borer JS, Kent KM, Maron BJ, Seides SF, Morrow AG, Epstein SE: Long-term hemodynamic and electrocardiographic assessment following operative repair of tetralogy of Fallot. Circulation 58(Suppl III):III-209, 1978.
56. Rowlatt UF, Rimoldi HJA, Lev M: The quantitative anatomy of the normal child's heart. Pediatr Clin North Am 10:499, 1963.
57. Stafford EG, Mair DD, McGoon DC, Danielson GK: Tetralogy of Fallot with absent pulmonary valve. Circulation 48(Suppl III):III-24, 1973.
58. Starr A, Bonchek LI, Sunderland CO: Total correction of tetralogy of Fallot in infancy. J Thorac Cardiovasc Surg 65:45, 1973.
59. Steeg CN, Krongrad E, Davachi F, Bowman FO Jr, Malm JR, Gersony WM: Postoperative left anterior hemiblock and right bundle branch block following repair of tetralogy of Fallot. Circulation 51:1026, 1975.
60. Stephenson LW, Friedman S, Edmunds LH: Staged surgical management of tetralogy of Fallot in infants. Circulation 58:837, 1978.
61. Sunderland CO, Matarazzo RG, Lees MH, Menashe VD, Bonchek LI, Rosenberg JA, Starr A: Total correction of tetralogy of Fallot: postoperative hemodynamic evaluation. Circulation 48:398, 1973.
62. Tucker WY, Turley K, Ullyot DJ, Ebert PA: Management of symptomatic tetralogy of Fallot in the first year of life. J Thorac Cardiovasc Surg 78:494, 1979.
63. Turley K, Tucker WY, Ebert PA: The changing role of palliative procedures in the treatment of infants with congenital heart disease. J Thorac Cardiovasc Surg 79:194, 1980.
64. Venugopal P, Subramanian S: Intracardiac repair of tetralogy of Fallot in patients under five years of age. Ann Thorac Surg 18:228, 1974.
65. Wolff GS, Rowland TW, Ellison RC: Surgically induced right bundle-branch block with left anterior hemiblock: an ominous sign in postoperative tetralogy of Fallot. Circulation 46:587, 1972.
66. Yabek SM, Jarmakani JM, Roberts NK: Diagnosis of trifascicular damage following tetralogy of Fallot and ventricular septal defect repair. Circulation 55:23, 1977.
67. Zavanella C, Matsuda H, Subramanian S: Successful correction of a complete form of atrioventricular canal associated with tetralogy of Fallot. J Thorac Cardiovasc Surg 74:195, 1977.

Transposition of the Great Arteries

23

Coauthored by Lucio Parenzan and Magdi Yacoub

The first approach to physiologic correction of transposition of the great arteries, based on transposing venous inflow, was conceived by Albert,[3] using animal experiments, and reported in 1954. Senning[64] reported in 1959 a successful intraatrial operation in humans utilizing the walls and septum of the atria. Shumacker[68] described in 1961 an operation using a bipedicled atrial flap. Mustard's report[47] in 1964 of an intraatrial transposition operation in a human using pericardium led to its almost universal use during the late 1960s and early 1970s. The 1970s saw a widespread return to the Senning operation in hopes of decreasing or eliminating some of the complications seen with the Mustard operation.[10,20,50,53]

Anatomic correction of transposition of the great arteries, based on transposing the great arteries and coronary arteries, was tried unsuccessfully as early as the 1950s.[7,32,36,48,64] Successful anatomic repair, reported by Jatene[35] in 1976 and Yacoub[87] in 1977, stimulated once again a strong interest in the possibilities of repair involving outflow correction, with its theoretical advantage of returning the left ventricle to the status of the systemic ventricle.

It is possible that the 1980s will see resolution of the many remaining questions regarding the proper choice of operation for transposition of the great arteries. Accurate and scientifically sound comparisons of the two commonly performed inflow operations—the Mustard and the Senning—should become available. As more patients who underwent inflow correction years ago enter their second postoperative decade there will be more information regarding the long-term ability of the right ventricle and tricuspid valve to function as the systemic ventricle and the systemic atrioventricular valve.

We will present in this chapter the three predominant operations for transposition of the great arteries in use today. The Mustard operation has always been our standard operation for transposition and will be presented as it is performed at the University of Oregon. The Senning operation will be presented as performed by Lucio Parenzan, Bergamo, Italy. The anatomic correction operation will be presented as performed by Magdi Yacoub, London, England.

Indications for Surgery

The outcome of transposition of the great arteries without intervention to increase systemic and pulmonary venous admixture is death for 80%–90% of infants by age 1 year.[51,65] This high mortality made search for an operative approach intense. A palliative procedure, atrial septectomy, was introduced by Blalock and Hanlon[13] in 1950. This was an effective means of increasing systemic oxygen saturation in a large proportion of patients, but was associated with a mortality of at least 20%–30%.[19,73]

Rashkind[54] introduced in the middle 1960s the technique of balloon atrial septostomy, performed by tearing the atrial septum with an inflated balloon at the tip of a catheter. This procedure was relatively easily performed in the catheterization laboratory, was quickly shown to result in improvement in most patients and to have a much lower mortality (approximately 10%) than the Blalock-Hanlon operation.[79] The Rashkind septostomy results in an adequate systemic arterial oxygen saturation (approximately 60%) in the majority of patients and short-term palliation, usually 6 to 12 months. At our institution a balloon septostomy is performed at the original catheterization in all patients with transposition of the great arteries. The balloon is usually passed at least eight times and inflated to 4 ml. Prostaglandin E_1 infusion is begun prior to catheterization if acidosis is present.[11]

Following performance of an atrial septostomy, there are two important questions that must be considered: (1) If the septostomy is unsatisfactory or is satisfactory for only a short time, what should the next step be—repeat septostomy, atrial septectomy, or correction? (2) What determines the timing of elective correction?

Failure of a Rashkind septostomy can occur because the atrial communication is not large enough or because the hemodynamic status is not conducive to intraatrial mixing. Although anatomic limitations can occur,[37] the more frequent cause of failure of a Rashkind septostomy is inadequate mixing in spite of an adequate septal opening. This is probably caused most frequently by unfavorable relative inflow resistances of the left and right ventricles and lack of the necessary streaming patterns.[42,58] The compliance or distensibility of the right ventricle is not low enough to permit adequate shunting from the left atrium to the right atrium.

This hemodynamic rather than physical cause of poor atrial mixing following a balloon septostomy explains the frequent lack of improvement if either a repeat septostomy or an atrial septectomy is performed.[88] Because an atrial septectomy is often not effective, we rarely perform it in a patient who has had a poor result from septostomy, but rather proceed to correction.

The timing of elective corrective surgery is based on the goal of performing it at an age and size associated with low risk and at the same time avoiding the morbid and mortal complications of transposition of the great arteries: (1) severe hypoxemia and acidosis, (2) cerebrovascular accident, and (3) development of pulmonary vascular disease. The frequency of these complications is demonstrated by a study of Gutgesell and colleagues[30] that showed a 14% incidence of death or cerebrovascular accident during the interval between septostomy and baffle repair.

The occurrence of cerebrovascular accidents and development of pulmonary vascular obstructive disease are time-related. Both are unusual in the first six months of life.[18,79] Development of pulmonary vascular obstructive disease is probably related to high hematocrit level and the resulting increase in resistance to pulmonary blood flow,[2] to the frequently increased pulmonary blood flow,[46] and to microthrombi.[49] Although rare, progressive pulmonary vascular disease can first be discovered after corrective operation, even in patients without preoperative evidence of pulmonary hypertension or elevated pulmonary vascular resistance.[12,38,49]

The proper timing of elective correction of transposition of the great arteries and intact ventricular septum appears to be between 6 and 12 months of age. Even earlier repair may be indicated, as suggested by Turley, Ebert, and co-workers,[77] who reported 34 infants repaired in the first 3 months of life with no operative mortality and a low incidence of late complications.

Choice of Corrective Operation

The choice of corrective operation involves these considerations: Should an inflow procedure (intraatrial switch) or an outflow procedure (anatomic correction or arterial switch) be chosen; and if an inflow procedure is chosen, which operation—the Mustard or Senning—is preferable?

The Mustard and Senning operations are the most popular procedures for venous transposition correction. Other inflow operations, such as the Baffes,[6] Shumacker,[4,68,81] and others,[5] have been described but have not been widely accepted.

The recent resurgence in popularity of the Senning operation reflects the persistence, in spite of many technical modifications, of the two main problems with the Mustard: atrial arrhythmias and venous obstruction. Although neither of these problems is necessarily major, they have caused many groups first to modify and then to abandon the Mustard in favor of the Senning.[10,20,50,53] At the same time other recent large series[77,78] of Mustard operations with excellent results have been reported, preventing any scientifically sound conclusion at the present time regarding which inflow operation is better.

Inflow operations are the most commonly performed procedures around the world for physiologic correction of transposition of the great arteries. This reflects the fact that they are relatively easily reproducible operations that can be performed by many surgeons with operative mortality below 10%. Nevertheless, long-term right ventricular function and long-term function of the tricuspid valve as the systemic atrioventricular valve are not known. The right ventricle does not appear to be structurally ideal for pumping against high resistance and is known to fail in many conditions that cause a high right ventricular pressure.

This concern for the potential long-term problems with inflow operations has stimulated development of operations to switch the arterial outflow, so that the left ventricle becomes the systemic ventricle.[70,84] Although such an operation was first performed in patients with preoperative systemic pressures in their left ventricle caused by the presence of a ventricular septal defect, it can be performed in patients with intact ventricular septum if the left ventricle is first "prepared" for a period of time by pulmonary artery banding.[87]

However, long-term problems may exist with anatomic correction. The anastomoses of the coronary arteries might not grow properly. The anastomosis of the aorta might not grow properly. The recurrence rate after resection and primary anastomosis for coarctation in infancy raises the possibility that there may be a similar problem with the ascending aortic anastomosis or the coronary anastomoses in anatomic correction.[25]

The gap between the proximal end of the transected aorta and the distal pulmonary artery almost always must be bridged by some prosthetic material. Although there is the hope that a sufficiently large tube to last through life can be used in infants, a second operation may well be necessary to place a larger pulmonary conduit.

The new aortic valve and its sinuses may not function normally without progressive dilatation and incompetence. There is always some discrepancy in size between the pulmonary arterial root and the ascending aorta. This abnormality in shape, combined with the thin arterial wall of the pulmonary artery, may lead to progressive dilatation later in life. An additional unknown is whether the left ventricle will maintain long-term normal function after correction.

Only time and careful follow-up of patients undergoing the various operations will answer the ultimate questions regarding choice of operation.

Surgical Strategy

Conduct of Cardiopulmonary Bypass

All operations in infants under 10 kg are performed using profound hypothermia and circulatory arrest (Chapter 5). In the case of inflow operations, the venous cannula is replaced in the right atrial appendage (the new left atrium) for venous drainage during rewarming. Cold crystalloid potassium cardioplegia is used for myocardial preservation (Chapter 6).

Management of Associated Defects

Ventricular Septal Defect

Ventricular septal defect occurs in approximately 20% of patients with transposition of the great arteries.[60] Pulmonary stenosis is also present in approximately 30% of patients with ventricular septal defects.[33]

Transposition with ventricular septal defect and no pulmonary stenosis is associated with very high mortality in infancy: most patients die before six months of age. Severe pulmonary vascular disease is common in survivors at one year of age. It is our practice to band the pulmonary artery in any patient with congestive heart failure that is not easily controlled by medical therapy. Subsequent corrective surgery is the Mustard operation, closure of the ventricular septal defect (usually through the tricuspid valve), and debanding of the pulmonary artery.[72,80]

There are other options available with transposition and ventricular septal defect. The Rastelli operation[44,55] may be performed: creation of a tunnel directing blood through the ventricular septal defect into the aorta, division of the pulmonary artery with oversewing of the proximal stump, and placement of an outflow conduit between the right ventricle and distal pulmonary artery. Another possibility is anatomic correction, including closure of the ventricular septal defect. Transposition with VSD and pulmonary vascular disease may be treated by a "palliative Mustard": a Mustard operation without closure of the VSD.[41,43]

Pulmonary Stenosis

Marked pulmonary stenosis is unusual in transposition with intact septum, occurring in less than 5%.[66,67] Some anatomic abnormality of the left ventricular outflow tract or small hemodynamic abnormality is common, reported in as many as 33% of patients.[60] The location of the stenosis can be at the valve, below the valve, or both.[8] Infants with severe pulmonary stenosis should undergo atrial septostomy and systemic-pulmonary shunt, with later repair at 2–3 years of age.

The approach to pulmonary stenosis at the time of correction is an area of controversy. The location and nature of the obstruction in the left ventricular outflow tract frequently defy successful repair by the direct approach.[55] Conduit bypass from the left ventricle to the pulmonary artery has been recommended.[21] Others,[9] however, recommend the direct approach, with excision of the muscular obstruction that is often present. Certainly, mild subvalvular stenosis may be left undisturbed and will not be of any consequence after a Mustard or Senning operation.

Patent Ductus Arteriosus
A large patent ductus arteriosus with high pulmonary blood flow is frequently lethal in the neonatal period. Such patients should probably undergo primary correction and ligation of the ductus.

Reoperation
Reoperation is sometimes necessary following the primary repair. Most reports deal with the problems that can occur with the Mustard operation: venous obstruction (systemic or pulmonary), residual ventricular septal defects, and patch leaks or dehiscence.[71,75]

An area of localized stenosis in the baffle can be repaired with a Dacron patch. Severe diffuse stenosis of the patch or dehiscence may require excision and replacement. Localized areas of detachment may be repaired. Residual ventricular septal defects can frequently be repaired through the tricuspid valve. Pulmonary venous obstruction can be corrected by patching the pulmonary venous atrium.[56]

Mustard Operation

Surgical Technique
The Mustard operation has the most variability of the three operations covered in this chapter. Among the variables are (1) atrial septal excision (amount and location),[40,78] (2) size and shape of the baffle,[1,52] (3) material of the baffle,[14,69,78] (4) position of the suture lines around the pulmonary vein and caval orifices,[78] (5) depth of the suture bites,[22] (6) incision of the coronary sinus,[22] (7) position of the patch in relation to the coronary sinus,[22] and (8) patching of the new left atrium (pulmonary venous atrium).[22,78] Because of these many variables, the Mustard operation may differ substantially from surgeon to surgeon.

Our technique of performing the Mustard operation is much like the original description by Mustard:[47] (1) the remaining atrial septum is excised, (2) the baffle is rectangular, (3) the baffle is autogenous pericardium, (4) the suture lines are close to the pulmonary venous orifices, but are somewhat away from the caval orifices, (5) the suture bites are relatively shallow, especially near the tricuspid valve, (6) the coronary sinus is left intact, (7) the patch is sutured so the coronary sinus drains with the systemic venous return, and (8) a patch is placed on the new left atrium (this differs from Mustard's original report).

Transposition of the Great Arteries

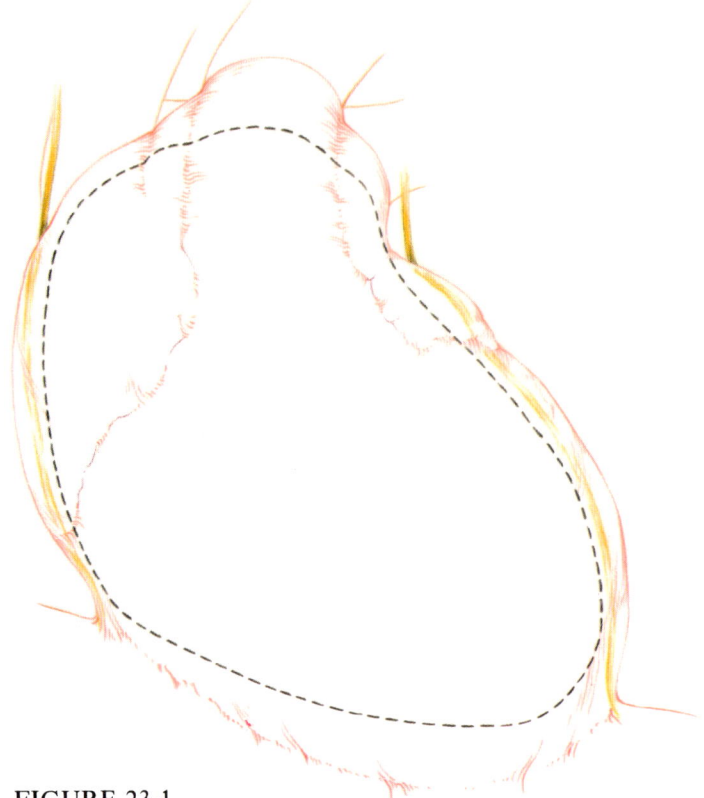

FIGURE 23-1

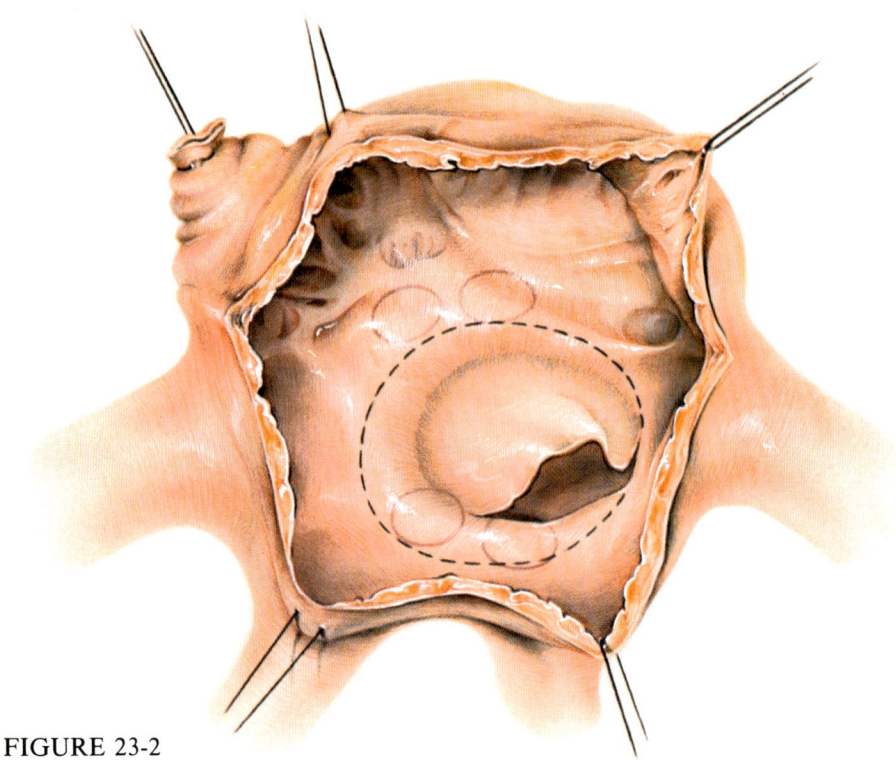

FIGURE 23-2

Pericardium is removed from phrenic nerve to phrenic nerve (Fig. 23-1). A rectangle is cut from the pericardium, to be used for the intraatrial baffle, and retraction sutures are placed in each corner. The remaining portion of pericardium is fashioned into a triangle to be used as the patch on the new left atrium (pulmonary venous atrium).

A longitudinal atriotomy is made in the right atrium just ventral to the caval-atrial junction. The edges of the right atrium are suspended.

The remaining atrial septum is excised (Fig. 23-2). The rim posteriorly over the right pulmonary veins, the rim inferiorly above the coronary sinus, the rim between the tricuspid and mitral valves, and the rim superiorly are excised, exercising caution to avoid cutting contiguous structures. The endothelium is reapproximated with interrupted 6-0 polyester sutures.

A retractor is placed over the atrial septum between the mitral and tricuspid valves, exposing the left atrium. The left pulmonary vein orifices and the base of the left atrial appendage are identified.

The first suture is then placed through the baffle and just on the left side of the carina between the left upper and lower pulmonary veins, and the suture is tied (Fig. 23-3). The superior suture line is brought laterally,

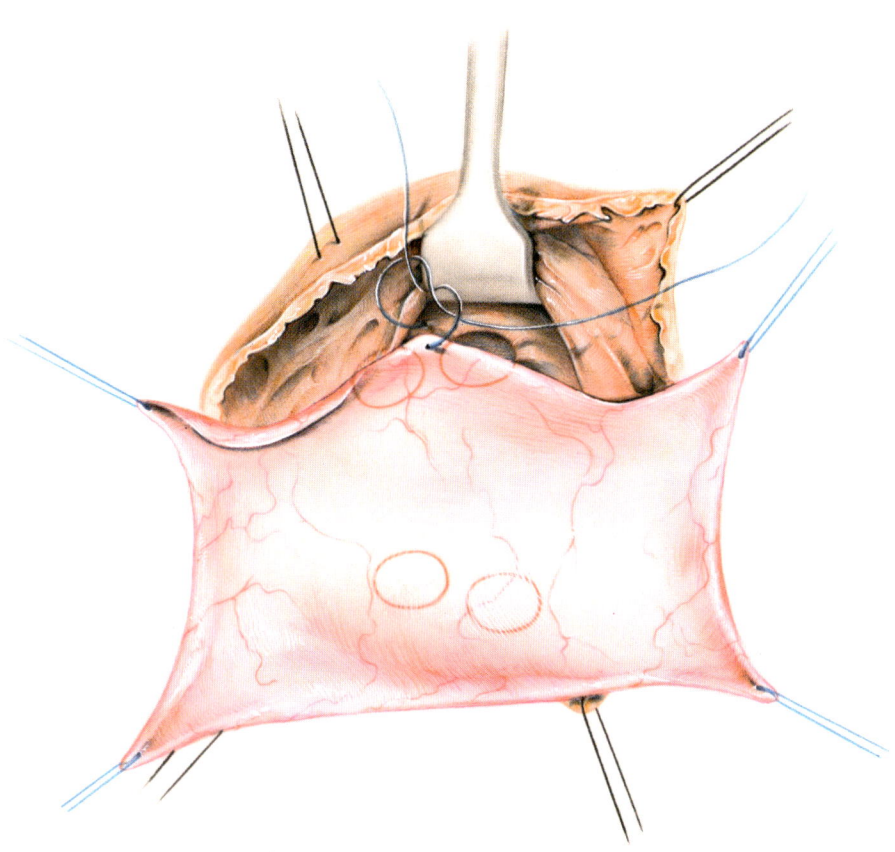

FIGURE 23-3

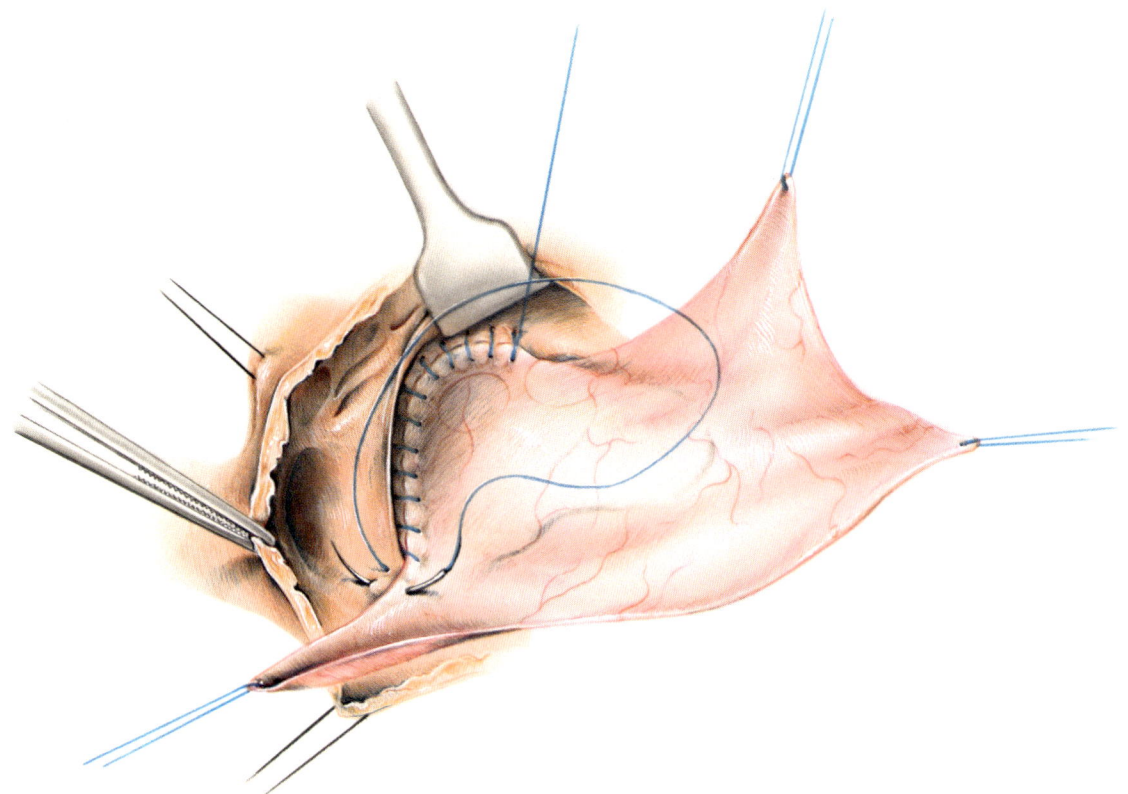

FIGURE 23-4

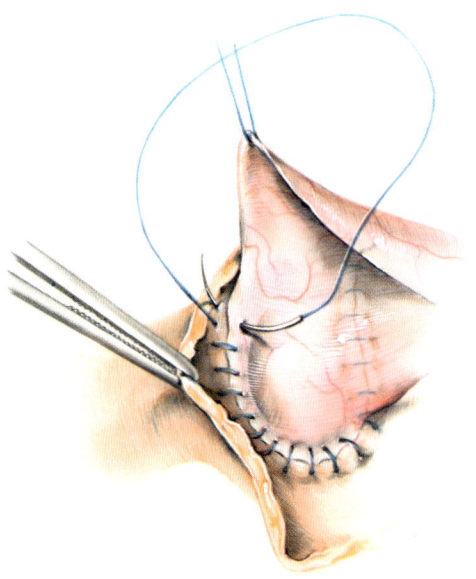

FIGURE 23-5

above the superior pulmonary veins, then below the superior vena cava orifice, 1–2 cm from the caval orifice (Fig. 23-4), around laterally and anteriorly, and tagged (Fig. 23-5).

The other end of the suture is brought inferiorly and laterally just below the inferior pulmonary veins (Fig. 23-6) and then around above the inferior vena cava orifice. This suture line should be parallel to the superior suture line until it reaches the lateral atrial wall.

As the suture line comes around the inferior vena cava orifice and anteriorly, the retractor is moved from over the atrial septum to within the right ventricle, through the tricuspid valve, and retracted anteriorly. This exposes the area of the coronary sinus and anterior atrial septum. The patch is then brought over and the shape is assessed. The suture line proceeds toward the anterior atrial septum, between the coronary sinus and the tricuspid valve

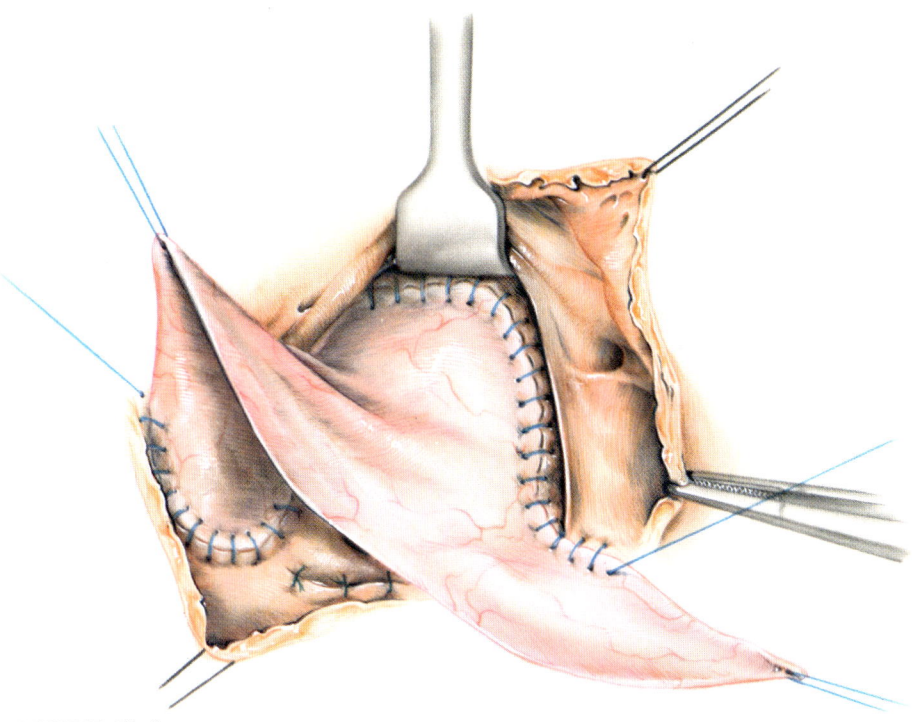

FIGURE 23-6

Transposition of the Great Arteries

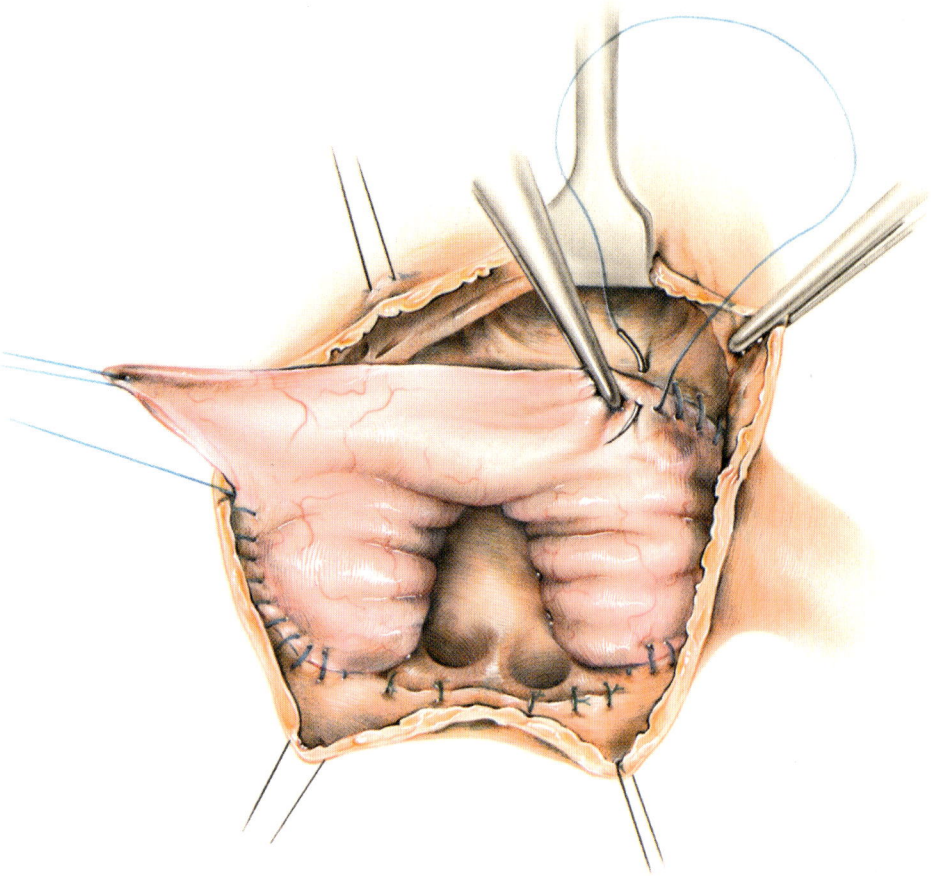

FIGURE 23-7

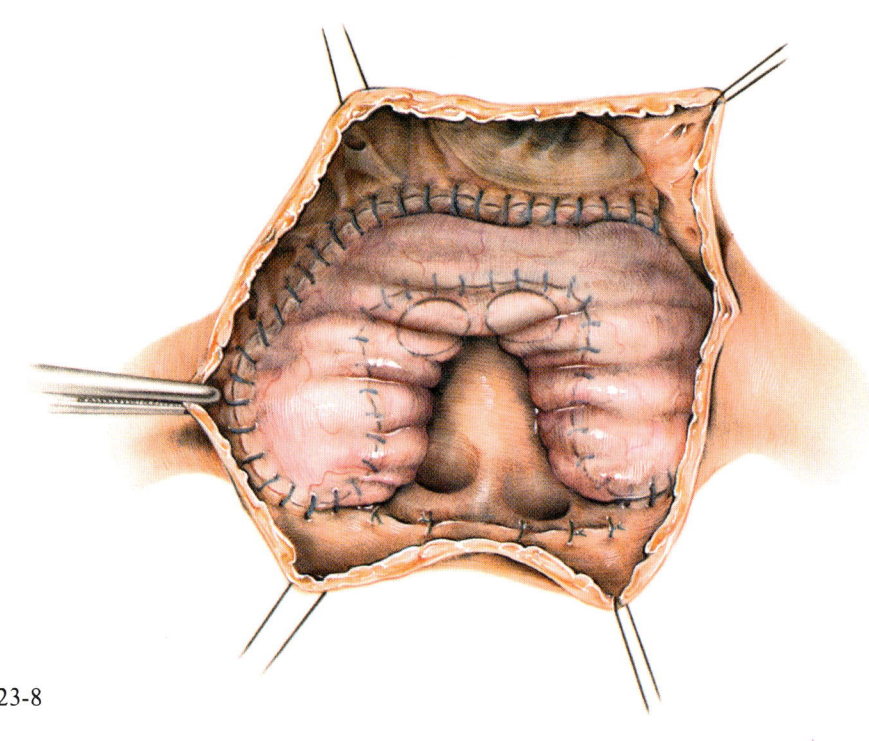

FIGURE 23-8

(Fig. 23-7), and goes across the remnant of atrial septum to complete the baffle suture (Fig. 23-8).

Cardioplegic solution is then injected into the aortic root to distend the baffle and thereby assess its configuration (Fig. 23-9). Any excessively redundant areas can be excised (Fig. 23-10).

The incision to enlarge the new left atrium is then made—down the lateral wall of the right atrium, through the ridge of the remnant of atrial septum, and between the right pulmonary veins (Fig. 23-11). The patch is then sutured from the inside (Fig. 23-12). The closure of the atriotomy incorporates the remaining side of the patch.

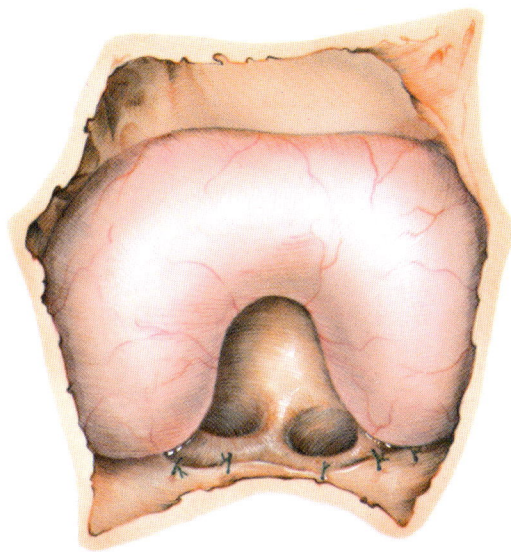

FIGURE 23-9

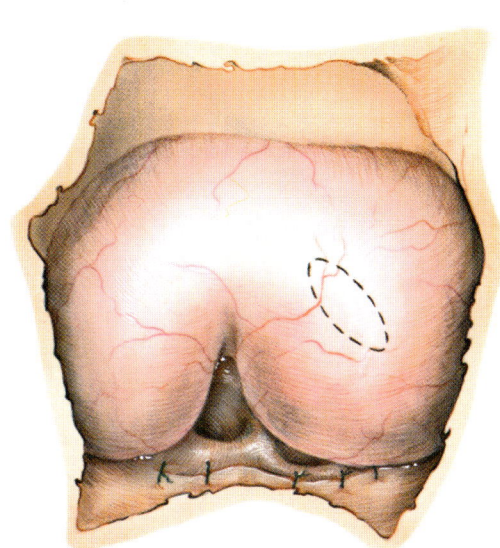

FIGURE 23-10

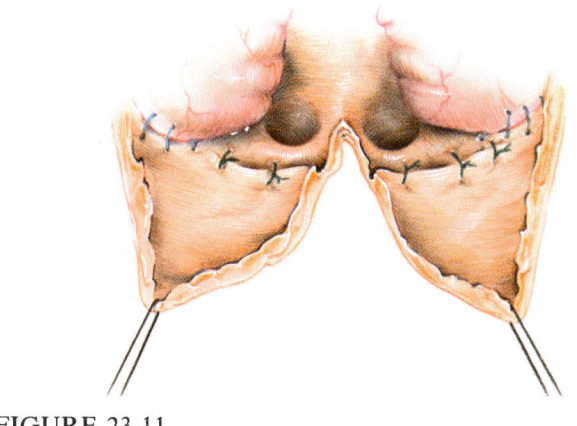

FIGURE 23-11

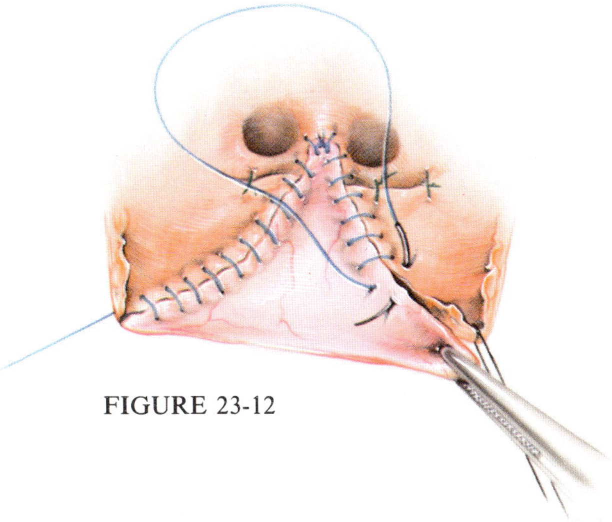

FIGURE 23-12

Results

Functional Status

Most patients, following the Mustard operation, have normal growth and normal physical activity.[15,31,39,74] Champsaur and colleagues[15] from the Hospital for Sick Children, Toronto, reported 91% of operative survivors were leading a normal life. Mustard's original patient was alive and well nine years after surgery. Symptoms or growth failure almost always indicates serious hemodynamic abnormalities.[40]

Electrophysiologic Changes

The following rhythms can occur following the Mustard operation:[16,23,24,26,29,31,34,59,61,83] (1) sinus rhythm, (2) a regular atrial rhythm appearing to originate in a location other than the sinus node, (3) atrial tachyarrhythmias and bradyarrhythmias, (4) junctional rhythm, and (5) atrioventricular block. There are often combinations of rhythms, usually with one predominating.[59] The incidence of arrhythmias as reported in the literature is influenced by the definition of what constitutes an arrhythmia and whether random electrocardiograms or 24-hour ambulatory monitoring is used for diagnosis. Inclusion of such minor arrhythmias as first-degree block can raise the incidence of arrhythmias to near 100%.[59,74] Holter monitoring for 24 hours also documents a higher incidence of arrhythmias.[59,78]

There is wide variation in the incidence of arrhythmias reported in the literature: sinus rhythm or a regular atrial rhythm from 63% to 97%;[15,59,76,78] junctional rhythm in up to 35%;[15,31,59] atrial flutter in as many as 6%;[15,59] and complete heart block in 0% to 3%.[15,59] The difference in the incidence of the various arrhythmias also appears to be related to variations in surgical technique.

There are three possible causes of rhythm disturbance following the Mustard operation: (1) injury to the sinus node or its artery, (2) interruption of atrial pathways, and (3) injury to the atrioventricular (AV) node. Opinions differ as to the relative importance of each factor.

It is clear that injury to the sinus node or its artery can cause arrhythmias.[16,23,24,26,27,61] El-Said and co-workers[23] have documented by histologic examination injury to the SA node, including hemorrhage early after operation and obliteration of the SA nodal artery and replacement of the SA node after longer postoperative periods. They have pointed out the importance of avoiding the area of the sinus node during cannulation. The sinus node can also be injured if the suture line is placed too near the superior caval orifice.[40,78]

The importance of the internodal or atrial preferential pathways is the subject of considerable debate. Isaacson and colleagues[34] concluded that extensive disturbance of the atrial septal connections between the sinus and atrioventricular nodes is frequently associated with serious dysrhythmia. This opinion is also held by Waldo[82] and Wittig.[83]

However, the importance of the internodal tracts is called into question by two facts: (1) electrophysiologic studies showing normal atrial conduction postoperatively[26] and (2) the high incidence of sinus rhythm even if no particular attention is paid to preservation of internodal tracts.[16,78] Gillette and co-workers[26] found no intraatrial block between the upper and lower intraatrial electrocardiograms in postoperative studies of patients in whom no special steps were taken to preserve internodal tracts. Ullal, Lincoln, and colleagues[78] report a very high incidence of sinus rhythm following their technique of performing the Mustard operation—a technique that almost certainly interrupts all three internodal tracts.

A disturbing fact is that sinus rhythm does not preclude disease of the sinus node, nor does it preclude the possibility of sudden death. Studies of sinus nodal recovery time have documented the fact that abnormal sinus nodal function can occur in the presence of sinus rhythm.[59] Approximately one-third of patients experiencing sudden death after the Mustard operation are in predominantly sinus rhythm prior to death.[62]

Hemodynamics

The physiologic results of the Mustard operation are influenced by the anatomic variations present at the time of operation, the variations in surgical technique, and the thoroughness of postoperative study. Thus, there is a broad range of reported postoperative hemodynamic results.

Table 23-1 (p. 110) lists a number of reports of postoperative catheterization findings in a total of 142 patients. There is wide variation in hemodynamic results: superior vena caval obstruction is present in 0%–54.5%, inferior vena caval obstruction in 0%–21.2%, pulmonary venous obstruction in 0%–33.3%, and baffle leaks in 0%–63.6%. During the mean intervals between operation and catheterization, which range from 10 months to 5.5 years, tricuspid valve function and right ventricular function have been good. Normal right ventricular function is present in over 90% of patients. Although some tricuspid insufficiency may occur in up to 40% of patients, it usually is present in less than 10%, and when present is mild and of no hemodynamic significance.

TABLE 23-1. Late Postoperative Hemodynamic Data After Mustard Operation

Authors	Number of Patients	Date of Report	Average Age at Surgery	Mean Interval Between Operation and Catheterization	Baffle Material	Superior Vena Caval Obstruction (over 5 mm Hg gradient)	Inferior Vena Caval Obstruction (over 5 mm Hg gradient)	Pulmonary Venous Obstruction	Baffle Leak	Tricuspid Insufficiency	Normal Right Ventricular Function
Clarkson et al.[17]	42	1976	Not given; range 11 days to 58 months	28 months	Pericardium	7.9%	0%	5.5%	0%	9%	100% (in patients with an intact septum)
Godman et al.[28]	14	1976	Not given; range 1.5 to 4.5 yr	5.5 yr	Pericardium	0%	0%	7.1%	35.7%	14%	93%
Hagler et al.[31]	33, all asymptomatic	1979	4.5 yr	4.7 yr	Dacron 73% Pericardium: 27%	27.3%	21.2%	12.1%	27.3%	42.4%	97%
Hagler et al.[31]	15, all symptomatic	1979	3.1 yr	1.7 yr	Dacron: 53% Pericardium: 47%	Total of 53.3%		33.3%	40%	40%	93%
Morgan et al.[45]	16	1972	Not given; range 5 months to 11 yr	10 months	Pericardium	6.3%	0%	Not evaluated	50%	11.1%	93%
Rodriguez-Fernandez et al.[57]	11	1972	Not given; range 2 to 7 yr	2.4 yr	Dacron: 55% Pericardium: 45%	9.1%	9.1%	0%	63.6%	Not studied	Not studied
Sunderland et al.[74]	11, all asymptomatic	1975	Not given; range 2.5 to 66 months	26 months	Dacron: 36% Pericardium: 64%	54.5%	0%	0%	36.4%	0%	100%

Senning Operation

This operation is performed today by most surgeons much as Senning originally described it in 1959.[64] Senning has subsequently described variations on his original technique.[63] The theoretical benefits of the Senning operation include (1) the use of atrial wall and interatrial septum, which will probably grow; (2) maintenance of atrial contraction; (3) possible decreased incidence of atrial arrhythmias; and (4) a more consistent and reproducible operation, since the dimensions of the baffle are determined by the dimensions of the atrium and interatrial septum and are therefore less variable than when pericardium is used.

Surgical Technique

The technique is essentially that of Senning[64] as modified by Quaegebeur, Brom, and colleagues.[53] The only foreign material is that used to enlarge the septal flap. Profound hypothermia with circulatory arrest is used. Hypothermic potassium-induced cardioplegia is the method of myocardial preservation.

The right atrium is incised longitudinally, a few millimeters ventral to the sulcus terminalis (Fig. 23-13). If a large eustachian valve is present, the incision is extended laterally to the base of the valve *(a)*. If the eustachian valve is small, the incision is extended more anteriorly *(b)*.

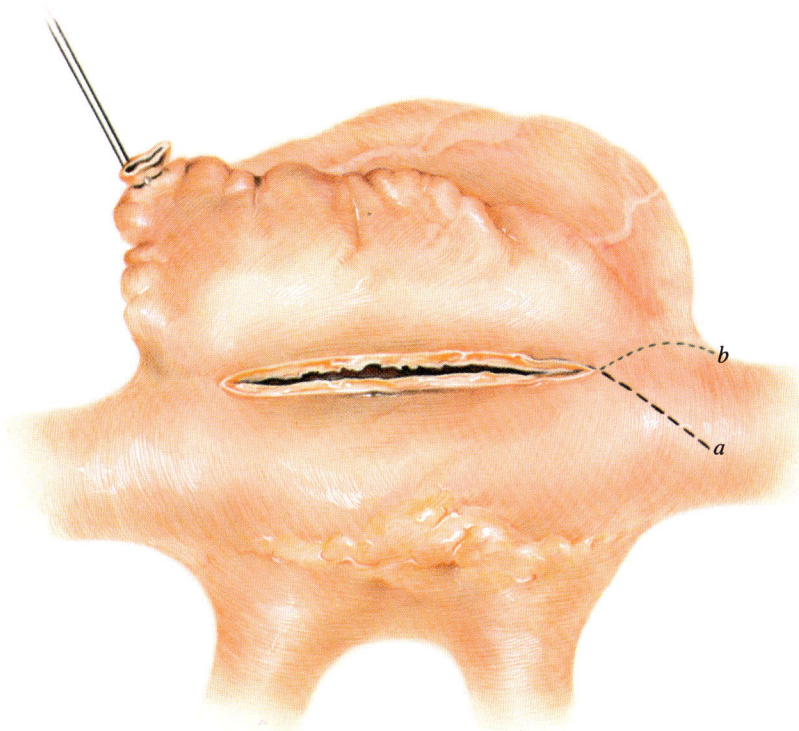

FIGURE 23-13

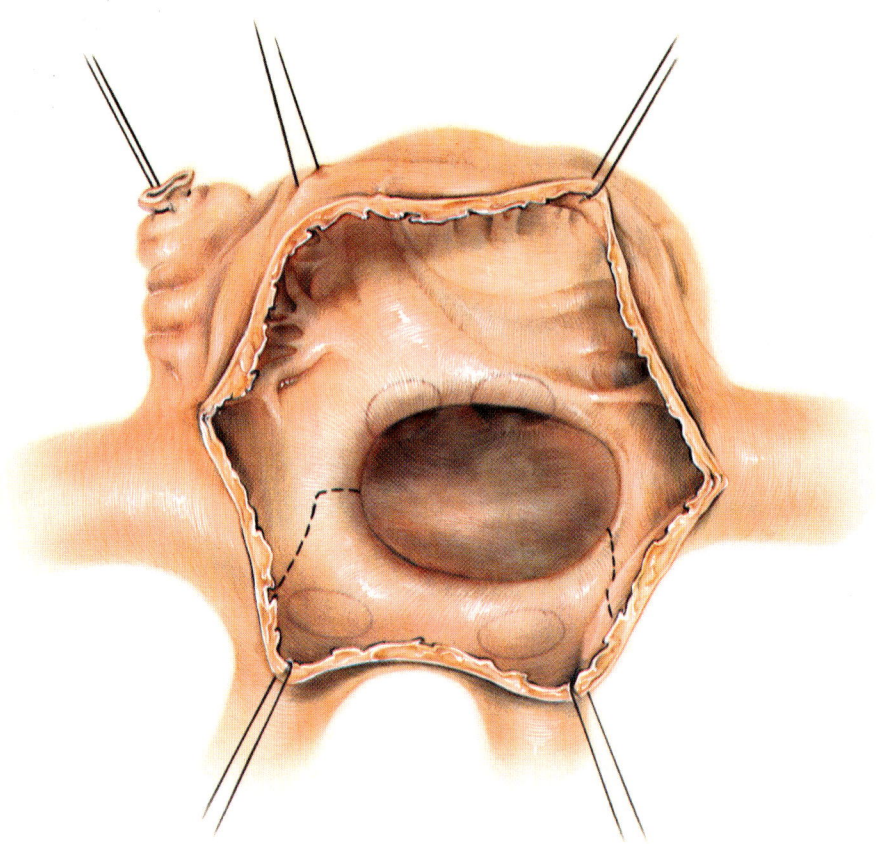

FIGURE 23-14

The atrial septum is incised to develop a trapezoid flap based at the interatrial groove (Fig. 23-14). This flap must be small so as to create a degree of rotation of the atrial edge when the flap is sutured over the pulmonary veins. The interatrial groove is dissected and the left atrium is opened by an incision (Fig. 23-15). This incision should not extend under either cava. The left atriotomy is enlarged by a short transverse incision between the right pulmonary veins.

The atrial flap is enlarged, if necessary, in the area of the foramen ovale, using Dacron. The flap is then sutured over the pulmonary veins (Fig. 23-16). The suture line begins between the left superior and inferior pulmonary vein orifices using running suture of 5-0 silk. The superior suture line is carried over the left superior pulmonary vein orifice and laterally and ends 1–2 cm below the superior vena caval orifice, at the base of the flap. The inferior suture line is also a running suture and proceeds around the inferior pulmonary vein orifice and laterally to the base of the flap, below the inferior vena caval orifice.

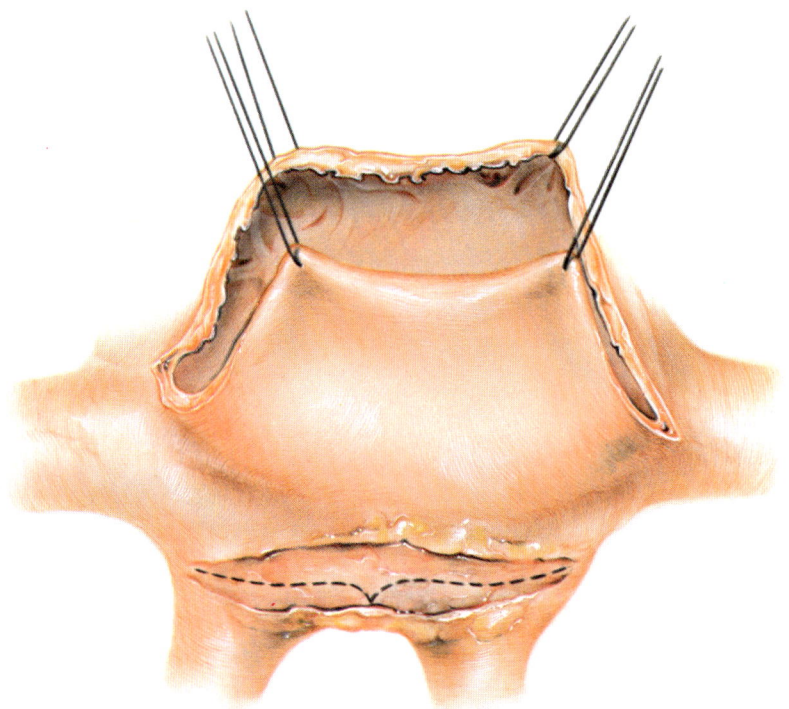

FIGURE 23-15

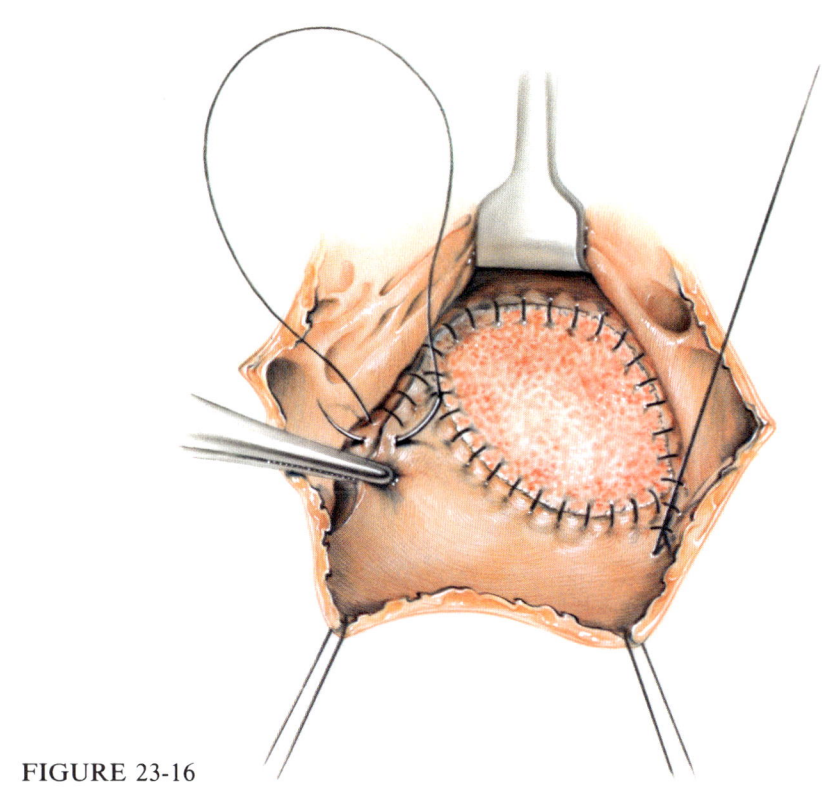

FIGURE 23-16

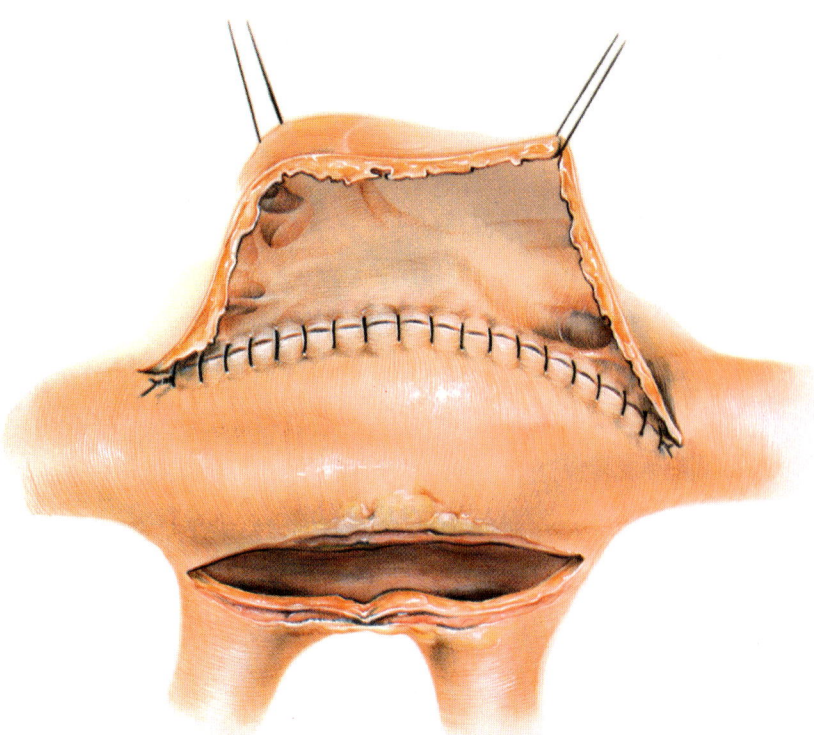

FIGURE 23-17

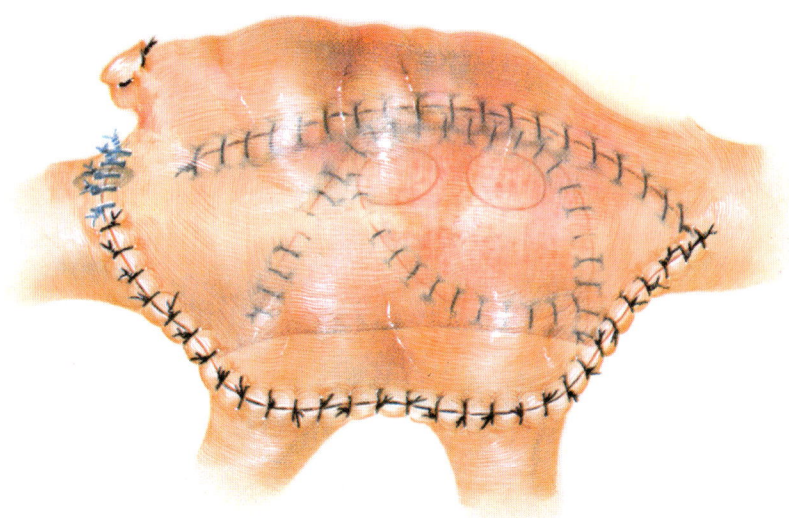

FIGURE 23-18

The dorsal edge of the right atrium is then sutured to the atrial septum between the tricuspid and mitral valves and over the orifices of the superior and inferior venae cavae, taking very small bites of tissue (Fig. 23-17). A multiholed cannula is placed through the left atrial appendage into the inferior vena cava, to stent the channel and later to drain blood from the inferior vena cava and atrium during rewarming. If a large eustachian valve is present, the inferior suture line incorporates the edge of the valve. The coronary sinus blood drains with the pulmonary venous blood.

The ventral edge of the right atrium is then sutured to the lateral edge of the left atriotomy and over the superior and inferior caval pathways (Fig. 23-18). Sutures are taken very superficially over the superior vena cava, using interrupted sutures of 6-0 polypropylene to avoid injury to the sinus node. The Senning repair creates overlying channels of venous inflow.

Results

Functional Status
Parenzan and co-workers[50] reported 24 patients, all of whom were asymptomatic.

Electrophysiologic Changes
Random electrocardiograms following the Senning operation show sinus rhythm in 83%–100%, junctional rhythm in 0%–17%, and atrioventricular block in 0%–4.7%.[20,50,53,64] One report[50] of 12 patients undergoing continuous 24-hour electrocardiograms showed constant sinus rhythm in 10 (83%) and 2 patients who had short episodes of junctional rhythm with rates above 80 beats per minute.

Hemodymanics
Senning[63] reported 44 patients with late follow-up, with only 1 case of superior vena caval obstruction and 1 case of pulmonary venous obstruction. Four reports[10,20,50,53] of postoperative catheterization studies total 40 patients. The incidence of caval obstruction was 0%. The incidence of pulmonary venous obstruction was 5% overall, but only occurred in one series.[20]

Anatomic Correction

Anatomic correction is the most theoretically appealing operation and the only operation that offers hope for complete correction of transposition of the great arteries, for the reasons covered earlier in this chapter. It is not commonly performed, however, because of the technical difficulties of transposing the coronary arteries, especially in small infants, and also because the majority of patients—those with intact septum—require the preliminary procedure of pulmonary artery banding to produce a left ventricle capable of pumping adequately against systemic resistance. These difficulties can be overcome with proper knowledge and experience, and the operation can be performed with an acceptably low risk.

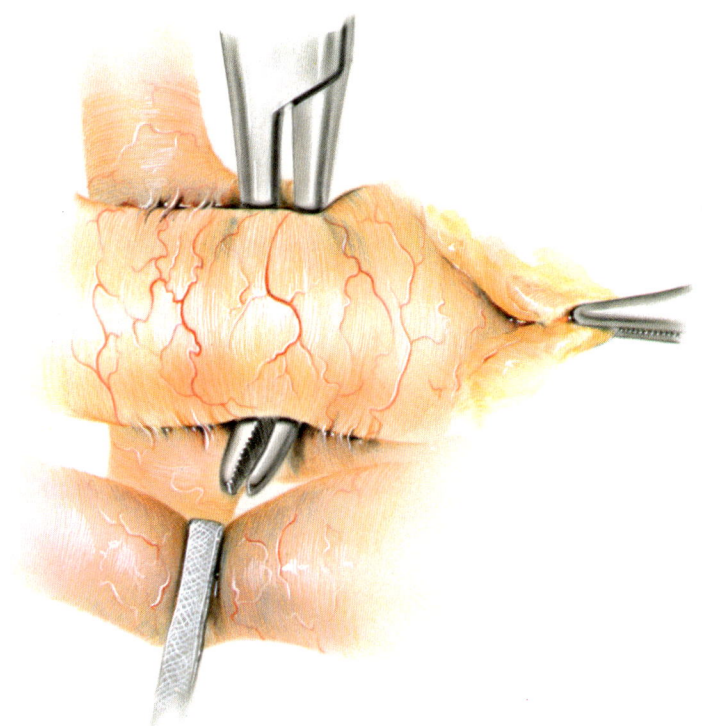

FIGURE 23-19

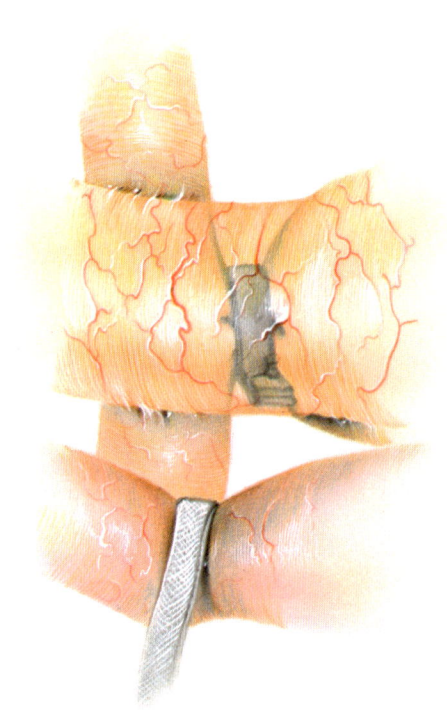

FIGURE 23-20

Preparation of the Left Ventricle

Anatomic correction can be performed as a one-stage procedure only in those patients with additional defects that result in systemic or near systemic pressure (at least two-thirds) in the left ventricle, such as ventricular septal defect, subpulmonary stenosis with normal pulmonary valve (any pulmonary valve abnormality is a contraindication to anatomic correction), or patent ductus arteriosus. After the first two weeks of life, all other patients require pulmonary artery banding, some in combination with a systemic-pulmonary shunt distal to the band, in order to maintain adequate pulmonary flow.

Banding is usually performed through a right anterolateral thoracotomy, since the main pulmonary artery is most accessible from this approach and a Blalock-Hanlon septectomy can be performed, if indicated, through the same approach.

A small opening is made between the aorta and pulmonary artery, in order to prevent migration of the band. The opening is made about 2 mm below the angle of the right and main pulmonary arteries, and the band is placed (Fig. 23-19). The band is adjusted (Fig. 23-20) to produce a proximal pressure near systemic and a distal pulmonary artery pressure that is pulsatile and has a systolic pressure of 15–20 mm Hg. Ventilation is temporarily stopped during measurement of distal pressure.

Banding alone is tolerated in the majority of patients; a small number with a relatively low total pulmonary flow require a systemic-pulmonary shunt. Low pulmonary flow is suspected preoperatively by a small cardiothoracic ratio (less than 0.55) and absence of pulmonary plethora on chest x-ray. At surgery, low pulmonary flow should be suspected if the pulmonary artery is relatively small compared with the aorta. If the diameter of the pulmonary artery is more than 1.2 times that of the aorta, a shunt is usually not necessary.

Low pulmonary flow is documented intraoperatively if banding results in a fall in arterial pO_2 of more than 10 mm Hg. If such a fall occurs, the band should be removed, a systemic-pulmonary shunt constructed distal to the position of the band, and the band replaced. A Blalock-Taussig shunt is preferred, since it leaves the aorta and main pulmonary artery unscarred. However, a polytetrafluoroethylene tube from the aorta to the main pulmonary artery may also be used.

Surgical Anatomy

An essential component of successful anatomic correction is transfer of the coronary arteries without kinking, torsion, or tension. This requires knowledge of the anatomic variations present in transposition and the ability to adjust technique to accommodate these variations.

The most common anatomy of the coronary arteries is origin from the right and left posterior sinuses of the aorta (type A, Fig. 23-21).[86] The second most common type is D, with the right coronary artery giving rise to the circumflex branch, which passes behind the pulmonary artery to reach the atrioventricular groove (Fig. 23-22). Both left and right coronary arteries can arise by a common trunk (type B, Fig. 23-23) or by two orifices in close proximity (type C, Fig. 23-24).

A fifth type, E (Fig. 23-25), is associated with the most rightward rotation of the aorta, with the arteries almost side by side. In this type the right coronary artery arises from the left coronary sinus and passes in front of the outflow tract of the right ventricle. Before doing so, it gives origin to the anterior descending coronary artery. The circumflex arises separately from the posterior sinus and curves behind the pulmonary artery to reach the atrioventricular groove.

Types A, D, and E are handled as illustrated in this chapter. Types B and C are managed by suturing the button containing the coronary ostium or ostia to the adjoining edge of the transected pulmonary artery. The distal end of the transected aorta is then fashioned to conform to the remaining circumference of the coronary artery button.

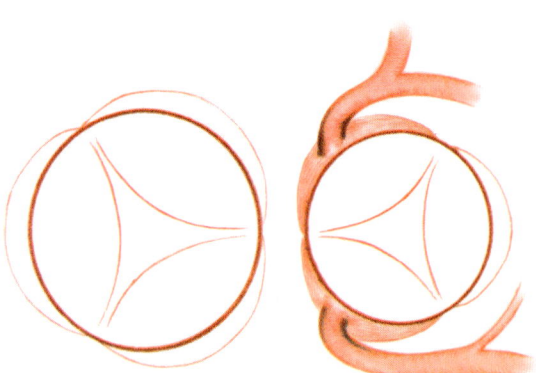

FIGURE 23-21. Type A.

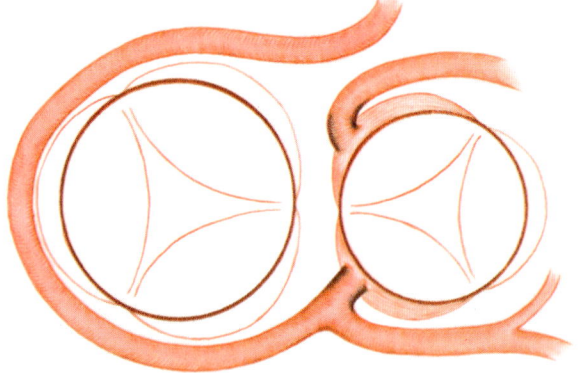

FIGURE 23-22. Type D.

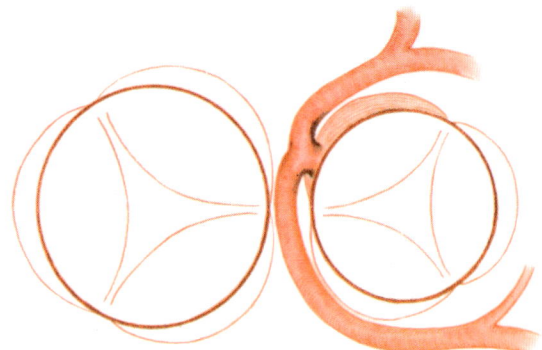

FIGURE 23-23. Type B.

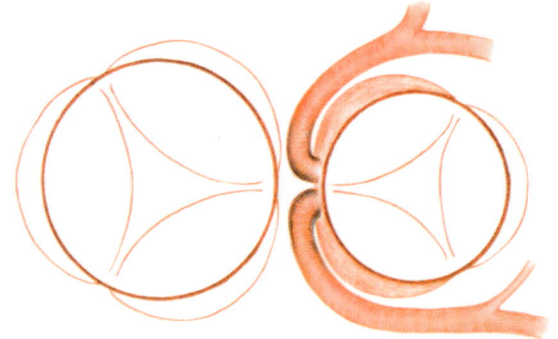

FIGURE 23-24. Type C.

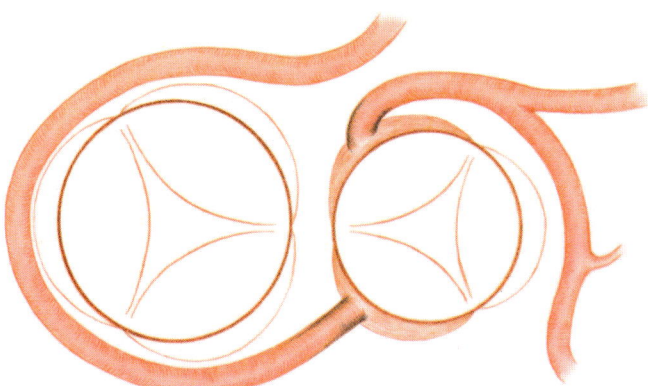

FIGURE 23-25. Type E.

Technique

The aortic cannula is placed as high as possible in the ascending aorta. The pulmonary artery is opened below the band, and the pulmonary valve and left ventricular outflow tract are inspected. As mentioned earlier, a normal pulmonary valve must be present to proceed with anatomic correction. The left ventricular outflow tract must either be normal or have easily correctable obstruction. If these conditions exist, the pulmonary artery is transected below the band and above the band, just below the bifurcation.

The coronary anatomy is assessed and marking sutures are placed on the pulmonary artery indicating the future position of the coronary ostia. The aorta is transected 1 mm above the top of the commissures (Fig. 23-26).

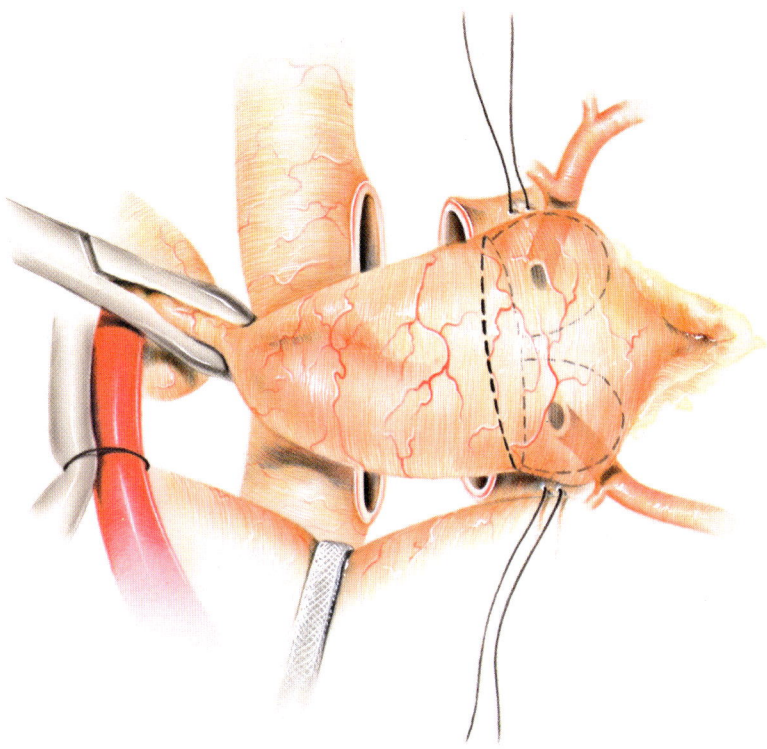

FIGURE 23-26

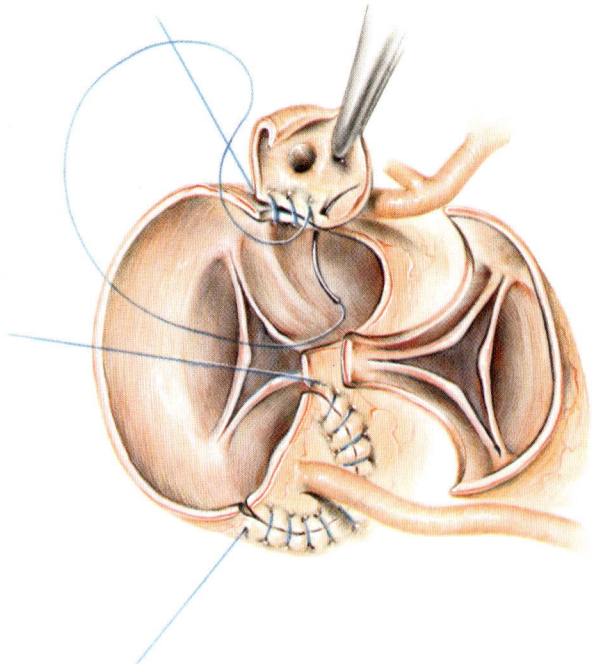

FIGURE 23-27

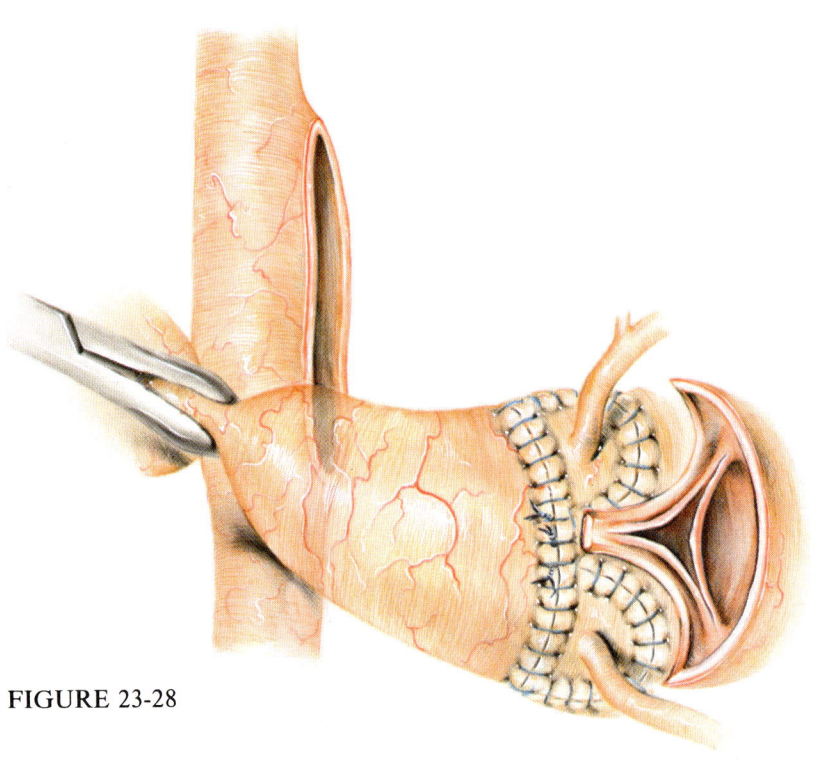

FIGURE 23-28

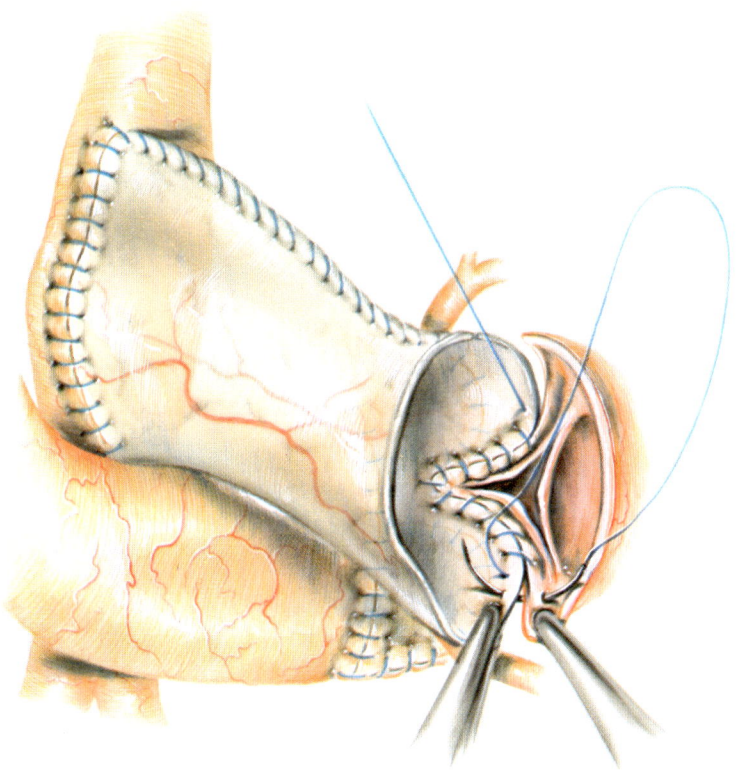

FIGURE 23-29

The coronary ostia are removed from the aorta, including most of the wall of the sinuses (Fig. 23-26). In type D the proximal portion of the circumflex coronary artery is dissected to provide mobility without kinking. Oval buttons are then cut from the pulmonary artery at the indicated points.

The coronary buttons are sutured to the pulmonary artery with 6-0 polypropylene (Fig. 23-27). The distal aorta is then connected with a triangular patch inserted to allow perfect approximation (Fig. 23-28), using 5-0 polypropylene. This patch is taken from the transected portion of pulmonary artery.

A pulmonary artery conduit is made of homologous dura mater that has been treated with antibiotic solution for 24 hours and stored in 95% glycerol. It is washed in saline for 15 minutes prior to use.

The pulmonary artery tube is usually about 25 mm in diameter and 45 mm in length. It is sutured with 5-0 polypropylene. Scallops are cut in the proximal portion and used to fill the defects in the sinuses (Fig. 23-29). The distal opening is enlarged as necessary by incising onto the branch pulmonary arteries. The conduit is usually placed to the patient's left side of the aorta.

The atrial septal defect is closed in standard fashion through a right atriotomy.

Results

Between 1976 and 1980, 19 patients with simple transposition of the great arteries, varying in age between 1 month and 2.5 years, underwent two-stage anatomic correction following a first-stage operation of pulmonary artery banding.[85] Correction was performed 5 weeks to 9 months (mean 3.9 months) later. There were 4 early (21%) and no late deaths.

Following an initial period of cardiac failure, all patients became asymptomatic with normal development. Repeat cardiac catheterization was performed in 9 patients. Left ventricular ejection fraction was normal in all; mild mitral regurgitation was present in 2, minimal aortic regurgitation in 5, and moderate supravalvar pulmonary stenosis in 1. The aortic and coronary anastomoses appeared to grow normally.

References

1. Aberdeen E, Waterston DJ, Carr I, Graham G, Bonham-Carter RE, Subramanian S: Successful correction of transposed great arteries by Mustard's operation. Lancet 1:1233, 1965.
2. Agarwal JB, Paltoo R, Palmer WH: Relative viscosity of blood at varying hematocrits in pulmonary circulation. J Appl Physiol 29:866, 1970.
3. Albert HM: Surgical correction of transposition of the great arteries. Surg Forum 5:74, 1954.
4. Alvarado A: Modified Shumacker operation for correction of transposition of the great arteries. J Thorac Cardiovasc Surg 74:614, 1977.
5. Angelini P, Sandiford FM: Functional correction of transposition of the great arteries: a new approach to avoid postoperative arrhythmias. J Thorac Cardiovasc Surg 66:86, 1973.
6. Baffes TG, Riker WL, DeBoer A, Potts WJ: Surgical correction of transposition of the aorta and pulmonary artery. J Thorac Cardiovasc Surg 34:469, 1957.
7. Bailey CP, Cookson BA, Downing DF, Neptune WB: Cardiac surgery under hypothermia. J Thorac Cardiovasc Surg 27:73, 1954.
8. Barcia A, Kincaid OW, Davis GD, Kirklin JW, Ongley PA: Transposition of the great arteries: an angiocardiographic study. Am J Roentgenol 100:249, 1967.
9. Barratt-Boyes BG: Discussion of Crupi et al. J Thorac Cardiovasc Surg 78:738, 1979.
10. Bender HW, Graham TP, Boucek RJ, Walker WE, Boerth RC: Comparative operative results of the Senning and Mustard procedures for transposition of the great arteries. Circulation 62(Suppl I):I-197, 1980.
11. Benson LN, Olley PM, Patel RG, Coceani F, Rowe RD: Role of prostaglandin E_1 infusion in the management of transposition of the great arteries. Am J Cardiol 44:691, 1979.
12. Berman W Jr, Whitman V, Pierce WS, Waldhausen JA: The development of pulmonary vascular obstructive disease after successful Mustard operation in early infancy. Circulation 58:181, 1978.
13. Blalock A, Hanlon CR: The surgical treatment of complete transposition of the aorta and the pulmonary artery. Surg Gynecol Obstet 90:1, 1950.
14. Breckenridge IM, Stark J, Bonham-Carter RE, Oelert H, Graham GR, Waterston DJ: Mustard's operation for transposition of the great arteries: review of 200 cases. Lancet 1:1140, 1972.
15. Champsaur GL, Sokol DM, Trusler GA, Mustard WT: Repair of transposition of the great arteries in 123 pediatric patients. Early and long-term results. Circulation 47:1032, 1973.
16. Clarkson PM, Barratt-Boyes BG, Neutze JM: Late dysrhythmias and disturbances of conduction following Mustard operation for complete transposition of the great arteries. Circulation 52:519, 1976.

17. Clarkson PM, Neutze JM, Barratt-Boyes BG, Brandt PWT: Late postoperative hemodynamic results and cineangiographic findings after Mustard atrial baffle repair for transposition of the great arteries. Circulation 53:525, 1976.
18. Clarkson PM, Neutze JM, Wardill JC, Barratt-Boyes BG: The pulmonary vascular bed in patients with complete transposition of the great arteries. Circulation 53:539, 1976.
19. Cooley DA, Hallman GL, Bloodwell RD, Leachman RD: Two-stage surgical treatment of complete transposition of the great vessels. Arch Surg 93:704, 1966.
20. Coto EO, Norwood WI, Lang PL, Castaneda AR: Modified Senning operation for treatment of transposition of the great arteries. J Thorac Cardiovasc Surg 78:721, 1979.
21. Crupi G, Anderson RH, Ho SY, Lincoln C: Complete transposition of the great arteries with intact ventricular septum and left ventricular outflow tract obstruction. J Thorac Cardiovasc Surg 78:730, 1979.
22. Ebert PA, Gay WA Jr, Engle MA: Correction of transposition of the great arteries: relationship of the coronary sinus and postoperative arrhythmias. Ann Surg 180:433, 1974.
23. El-Said GM, Gillette PC, Cooley DA, Mullins CE, Williams RL, McNamara DG: Protection of the sinus node in Mustard's operation. Circulation 53:788, 1976.
24. El-Said G, Rosenberg HS, Mullins CE, Hallman GL, Cooley DA, McNamara DG: Dysrhythmias after Mustard's operation for transposition of the great arteries. Am J Cardiol 30:526, 1972.
25. Fleming WH: Why switch? J Thorac Cardiovasc Surg 78:1, 1979.
26. Gillette PC, El-Said GM, Sivarajan N, Mullins CE, Williams RL, McNamara DG: Electrophysiological abnormalities after Mustard's operation for transposition of the great arteries. Br Heart J 36:186, 1974.
27. Gillette PC, Kugler JD, Garson A Jr, Gutgesell HP, Duff DF, McNamara DG: Mechanisms of cardiac arrhythmias after the Mustard operation for transposition of the great arteries. Am J Cardiol:45:1225, 1980.
28. Godman MJ, Friedli B, Pasternac A, Kidd BSL, Trusler GA, Mustard WT: Hemodynamic studies in children four to ten years after the Mustard operation for transposition of the great arteries. Circulation 53:532, 1976.
29. Greenwood RD, Rosenthal A, Sloss LJ, LaCorte M, Nadas AS: Sick sinus syndrome after surgery for congenital heart disease. Circulation 52:208, 1975.
30. Gutgesell HP, Garson A, McNamara DG: Prognosis for the newborn with transposition of the great arteries. Am J Cardiol 44:96, 1979.
31. Hagler DJ, Ritter DG, Mair DD, Tajik AJ, Seward JB, Fulton RE, Ritman EL: Right and left ventricular function after the Mustard procedure in transposition of the great arteries. Am J Cardiol 44:276, 1979.
32. Idriss FS, Goldstein IR, Grana L, French D, Potts WJ: A new technic for complete correction of transposition of the great vessels. Circulation 24:5, 1961.
33. Imamura ES, Morikawa T, Tatsumo K, Konno S, Arai T, Sakakibara S: Surgical considerations of ventricular septal defect associated with complete transposition of the great arteries and pulmonary stenosis: with special reference to the Rastelli operation. Circulation 45:914, 1971.
34. Isaacson R, Titus JL, Merideth J, Feldt RH, McGoon DC: Apparent interruption of atrial conduction pathways after surgical repair of transposition of great arteries. Am J Cardiol 30:533, 1972.
35. Jatene AD, Fontes VF, Paulista PP, Souza LCB, Neger F, Galantier M, Sousa JEMR: Anatomic correction of transposition of the great vessels. J Thorac Cardiovasc Surg 72:364, 1976.
36. Kay EB, Cross FS: Surgical treatment of transposition of the great vessels. Surgery 38:712, 1955.
37. Korns ME, Garabedian HA, Lauer RM: Anatomic limitations of balloon atrial septostomy. Hum Pathol 3:345, 1972.
38. Lakier JB, Stanger P, Heymann MA, Hoffman JIE, Rudolph AM: Early onset

of pulmonary vascular obstruction in patients with aortopulmonary transposition and intact septum. Circulation 51:875, 1975.
39. Levy RJ, Rosenthal A, Castaneda AR, Nadas AS: Growth after surgical repair of simple d-transposition of the great arteries. Ann Thorac Surg 25:225, 1978.
40. Lewis AB, Lindesmith GG, Takahashi M, Stanton RE, Tucker BL, Stiles QR, Meyer BW: Cardiac rhythm following the Mustard procedure for transposition of the great vessels. J Thorac Cardiovasc Surg 73:919, 1977.
41. Lindesmith GC, Stiles QR, Tucker BL, Gallaher ME, Stanton RE, Meyer BW: The Mustard operation as a palliative procedure. J Thorac Cardiovasc Surg 63:75, 1972.
42. Mair DD, Ritter DG: Factors influencing intracirculatory mixing in patients with complete transposition of the great arteries. Am J Cardiol 30:653, 1972.
43. Mair DD, Ritter DG, Danielson GK, Wallace RB, McGoon DC: The palliative Mustard operation. Rationale and results. Am J Cardiol 37:762, 1976.
44. McGoon DC, Wallace RB, Danielson GK: The Rastelli operation. J Thorac Cardiovasc Surg 65:65, 1973.
45. Morgan JR, Miller BL, Daicoff GR, Andrews EJ: Hemodynamic and angiocardiographic evaluation after Mustard procedure for transposition of the great arteries. J Thorac Cardiovasc Surg 64:878, 1972.
46. Murray JF, Karp RB, Nadel JA: Viscosity effects on pressure-flow relations and vascular resistance in dogs' lungs. J Appl Physiol 27:336, 1969.
47. Mustard WT: Successful two-stage correction of transposition of the great vessels. Surgery 55:469, 1964.
48. Mustard WT, Chute AL, Keith JD, Sirek A, Rowe RD, Vlad P: A surgical approach to transposition of great vessels with extracorporeal circuit. Surgery 36:39, 1954.
49. Newfeld EA, Paul MH, Muster AJ, Idriss FS: Pulmonary vascular disease in complete transposition of the great arteries: a study of 200 patients. Am J Cardiol 34:75, 1974.
50. Parenzan L, Locatelli G, Alfieri O, Villani M, Invernizzi G: The Senning operation for transposition of the great arteries. J Thorac Cardiovasc Surg 76:305, 1978.
51. Paul MH: D-transposition of the great arteries. *In* Moss A, Adams F, Emmanouilides G (eds): Heart Diseases in Infants, Children, and Adolescents. Baltimore, Williams & Wilkins, 1978, p 301.
52. Quaegebeur JM, Brom AG: The trousers-shaped baffle for use in the Mustard operation. Ann Thorac Surg 25:240, 1978.
53. Quaegebeur J, Rohmer J, Brom AG: Revival of the Senning operation in the treatment of transposition of the great arteries. Thorax 32:517, 1977.
54. Rashkind WJ, Miller WW: Creation of an atrial septal defect without thoracotomy. JAMA 196:991, 1966.
55. Rastelli GC, Wallace RB, Ongley PA: Complete repair of transposition of the great arteries with pulmonary stenosis: a review and report of a case corrected by using a new surgical technique. Circulation 39:83, 1969.
56. Reul GJ, Cooley DA, Sandiford FM, Hallman GL: Complications following the contoured Dacron baffle in correction of transposition of the great arteries. Surgery 76:946, 1974.
57. Rodriguez-Fernandez HL, Kelly DT, Collado A, Haller A, Krovetz LJ, Rowe RD: Hemodynamic data and angiographic findings after Mustard repair for complete transposition of the great arteries. Circulation 47:799, 1972.
58. Rudolph AM: Congenital Diseases of the Heart. Chicago, Year Book Medical Publishers, 1974, p 245.
59. Saalouke MG, Rios J, Perry LW, Shapiro SR, Scott LP: Electrophysiologic studies after Mustard's operation for d-transposition of the great vessels. Am J Cardiol 41:1104, 1978.
60. Sansa M, Tonkin IL, Bargeron LM Jr, Elliott LP: Left ventricular outflow tract obstruction in transposition of the great arteries: an angiographic study of 74 cases. Am J Cardiol 44:88, 1979.

61. Schraut W, Lin CY, de la Fuente D, Arcilla R, Replogle RL: Avoiding postoperative dysrhythmias and venous obstruction following Mustard's operation. Ann Thorac Surg 18:142, 1974.
62. Scott LP, Saalouke MG, Shapiro SR, Rios JC, Perry LW: Sudden unexpected death following Mustard's procedure for d-transposition of the great vessels (abstr). Circulation 54(Suppl II):II-89, 1976.
63. Senning A: Correction of the transposition of the great arteries. Ann Surg 182:287, 1975.
64. Senning A: Surgical correction of transposition of the great vessels. Surgery 45:966, 1959.
65. Shaher RM: Complete Transposition of the Great Arteries. New York, Academic Press, 1973, p 409.
66. Shaher RM, Moes CAF, Khoury G: Radiologic and angiocardiographic findings in complete transposition of the great vessels with left ventricular outflow tract obstruction. Radiology 88:1092, 1967.
67. Shaher RM, Puddu GC, Khoury G, Moes CAF, Mustard WT: Complete transposition of the great vessels with anatomic obstruction of the outflow tract of the left ventricle. Surgical implications of anatomic findings. Am J Cardiol 19:658, 1967.
68. Shumacker HB Jr: A new operation for transposition of the great vessels. Surgery 50:773, 1961.
69. Stafford EG, McGoon DC: The Mustard operation. Mayo Clin Proc 48:119, 1973.
70. Stansel HC Jr: A new operation for d-loop transposition of the great vessels. Ann Thorac Surg 19:565, 1975.
71. Stark J, Tynan MJ, Ashcraft KW, Aberdeen E, Waterston DJ: Obstruction of pulmonary veins and superior vena cava after the Mustard operation for transposition of the great arteries. Circulation 45, 46(Suppl I):I-116, 1972.
72. Stark J, Tynan M, Tatooles CJ, Aberdeen E, Waterston JD: Banding of the pulmonary artery for transposition of the great arteries and ventricular septal defect. Circulation 41,42(Suppl II):II-116, 1970.
73. Starr A, Campbell TJ, Wood J, McCord C, Herr R, Menashe V: Transposition of the great vessels: recent experience with the Blalock-Hanlon procedure. Am J Surg 108:198, 1964.
74. Sunderland CO, Henken DP, Nichols GM, Dhindsa DS, Bonchek LI, Menashe VD, Rahimtoola SH, Starr A: Postoperative hemodynamic and electrophysiologic evaluation of the interatrial baffle procedure. Am J Cardiol 35:660, 1975.
75. Szarnicki RJ, Stark J, de Leval M: Reoperation for complications after inflow correction of transposition of the great arteries: technical considerations. Ann Thorac Surg 25:150, 1978.
76. Turley K, Ebert PA: Total correction of transposition of the great arteries: conduction disturbances in infants younger than three months of age. J Thorac Cardiovasc Surg 76:312, 1978.
77. Turley K, Vinocur B, Heymann M, Rudolph A, Ebert PA: Intraatrial repair of transposition of the great arteries in infancy, early and late results (abstr). Am J Cardiol 45:448, 1980.
78. Ullal RR, Anderson RH, Lincoln C: Mustard's operation modified to avoid dysrhythmias and systemic venous obstruction. J Thorac Cardiovasc Surg 78:431, 1979.
79. Vlad P, Lambert EC: Late results of Rashkind's balloon atrial septostomy in transposition. *In* Kirklin JW (ed): Advances in Cardiovascular Surgery. New York, Grune & Stratton, 1973, pp 29–36.
80. Waldhausen JA, Boruchow I, Miller WW, Rashkind WJ: Transposition of the great arteries with ventricular septal defect: palliation by atrial septostomy and pulmonary artery banding. Circulation 39,40(Suppl I):I-215, 1969.
81. Waldhausen JA, Pierce WS, Berman W Jr, Whitman V: Modified Shumacker repair of transposition of the great arteries. Circulation 60(Suppl I):I-110, 1979.

82. Waldo AL, Krongrad E, Bowman FO, Kaiser GA, Husson GS, Malm JR: Electrophysiological considerations during total repair of transposition of the great vessels. Circulation 46(Suppl II):II-34, 1972.
83. Wittig JH, de Leval MR, Stark J: Intraoperative mapping of atrial activation before, during, and after the Mustard operation. J Thorac Cardiovasc Surg 73:1, 1977.
84. Yacoub MH: The case for anatomic correction of transposition of the great arteries. J Thorac Cardiovasc Surg 78:3, 1979.
85. Yacoub M, Bernhard A, Lange P, Radley-Smith R, Keck E. Stephan E, Heintzen P: Clinical and hemodynamic results of the two-stage anatomic correction of simple transposition of the great arteries. Circulation 62(Suppl I):I-190, 1980.
86. Yacoub MH, Radley-Smith R: Anatomy of the coronary arteries in transposition of the great arteries and methods for their transfer in anatomical correction. Thorax 33:418, 1978.
87. Yacoub MH, Radley-Smith R, Maclaurin R: Two-stage operation for anatomical correction of transposition of the great arteries with intact interventricular septum. Lancet 1:1275, 1977.
88. Zavanella C, Subramanian S: Review: surgery for transposition of the great arteries in the first year of life. Ann Surg 187:143, 1978.

Total Anomalous Pulmonary Venous Connection

Total anomalous pulmonary venous connection (TAPVC) can be supracardiac, cardiac, infracardiac, or mixed. A variety of surgical approaches have been described. Management has become more standardized during the past decade, and excellent results can be achieved.

Indications for Surgery

Patients with TAPVC usually present with severe cyanosis and/or pulmonary edema as infants, often within the first days or weeks of life.[2,5,12] Infracardiac type usually presents within the first month of life, the other types usually within the first three months. The natural history is death for 80% of symptomatic infants before age one year.[2]

The grave prognosis of medical management makes surgery the treatment of choice in almost all cases. Although balloon atrial septostomy and delay of surgery has been recommended,[22,33] such is not our policy. Surgery should be performed in symptomatic patients regardless of age or size.[16,29,31]

Surgical Strategy

Infants are operated upon using profound hypothermia and circulatory arrest (Chapter 5) with cold potassium crystalloid cardioplegia (Chapter 6) for myocardial preservation.

Supracardiac Type

Supracardiac TAPVC is the most common type, accounting for approximately one-half of cases.[29,33]

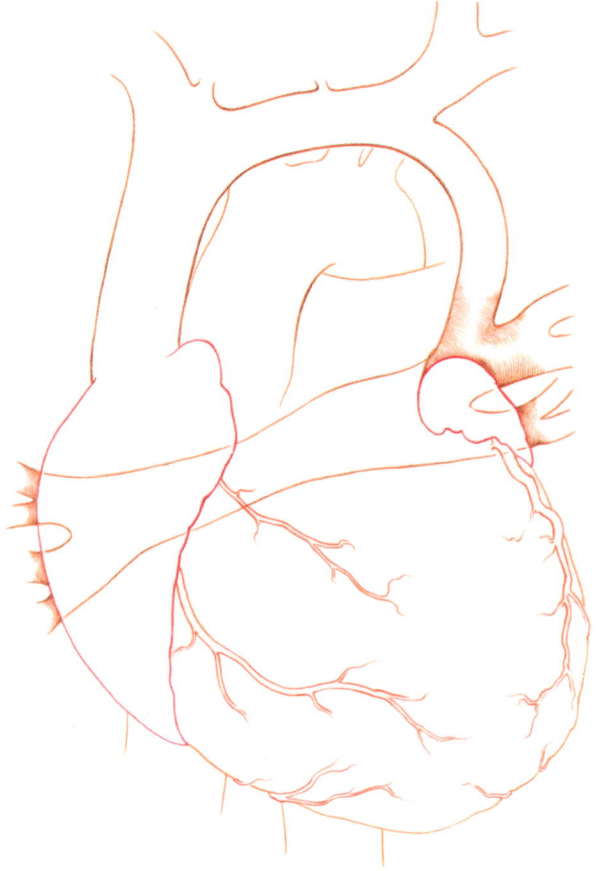

FIGURE 24-1

Surgical Anatomy

The pulmonary veins join a transverse pulmonary venous trunk (Fig. 24-1). The pulmonary venous trunk is usually connected to the innominate vein by a left vertical vein. In rare instances, the connection may be to the superior vena cava. There is a foramen ovale atrial septal defect.

The left atrium is frequently small, although the appendage is usually of normal size.[20] This may limit ventricular filling and cardiac performance in the postoperative period.[24] The left ventricular chamber may also be small.[1,3,4]

Surgical Technique

Muller[21] reported partial correction of supracardiac TAPVC in 1951 using a closed technique for side-to-side anastomosis of the pulmonary venous trunk and left atrium. The first successful complete correction, using cardiopulmonary bypass, was reported by Cooley and Ochsner[7] in 1957. Many approaches to correction have been described, including (1) median sternotomy with repair through the right atrium,[7] (2) left posterolateral thoracotomy,[25,26] (3) median sternotomy with transverse incision through the right atrium into the left atrium and extension of the anastomosis onto the right atrial wall,[27] (4) median sternotomy with elevation and retraction of the cavae to the left and construction of the anastomosis from the right side,[19] (5) median sternotomy with elevation of the apex toward the patient's right shoulder and construction of the anastomosis behind the heart,[6,32] and (6) median sternotomy with anastomosis through the transverse sinus.[28] We prefer elevating the apex (method 5), since this method allows extension of the anastomosis into the left upper vein if necessary.

Following circulatory arrest and injection of cold cardioplegic solution, the apex is elevated, exposing the posterior pericardium and the pulmonary venous trunk. The pericardium is incised (Fig. 24-2), exposing the venous trunk and the connection of the left vertical vein. The left vertical vein is encircled and tied (Fig. 24-3). Incisions are then made in the venous trunk and the left atrium (Fig. 24-4). If the left atrium is very small the incision is extended onto the appendage.

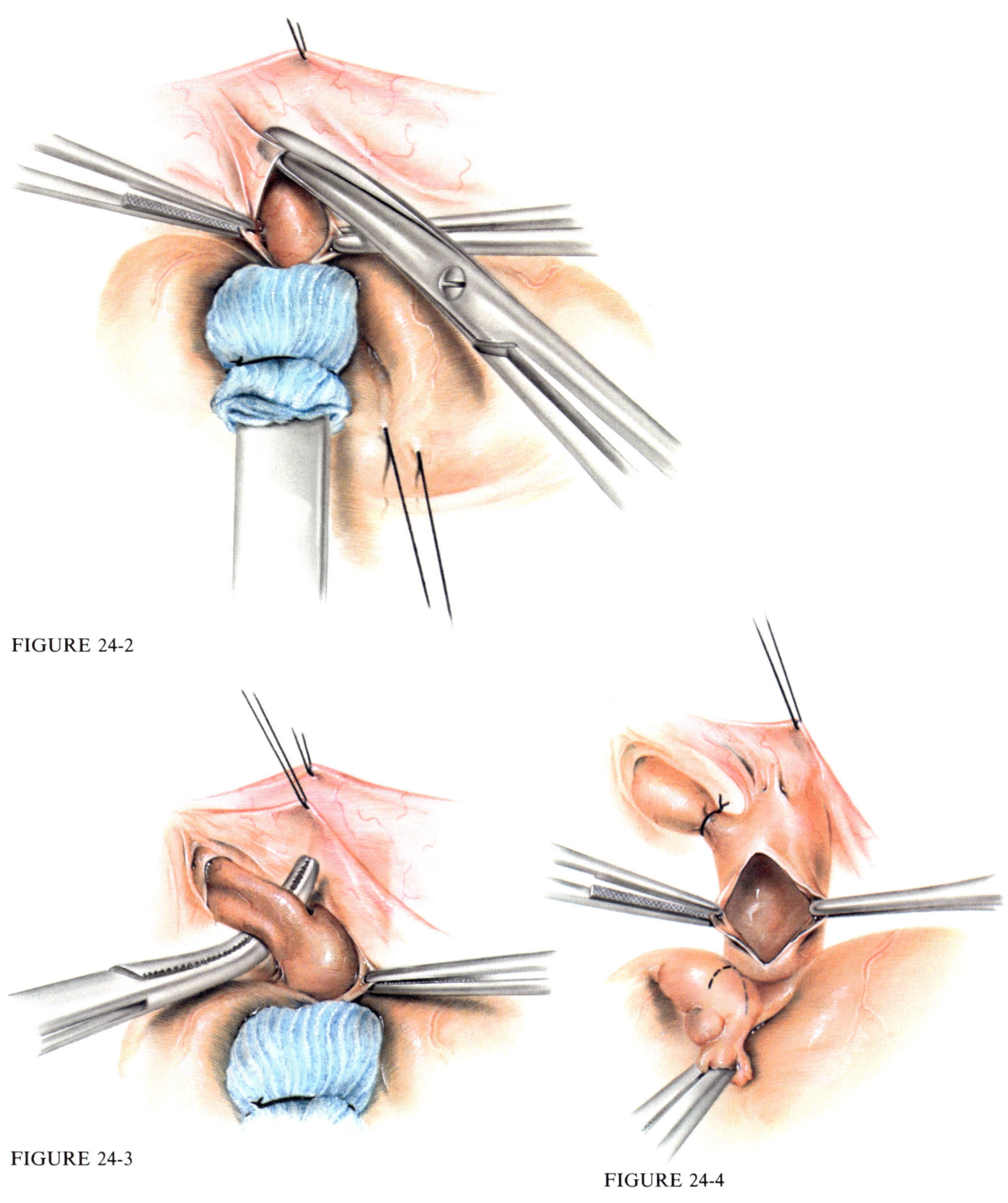

FIGURE 24-2

FIGURE 24-3

FIGURE 24-4

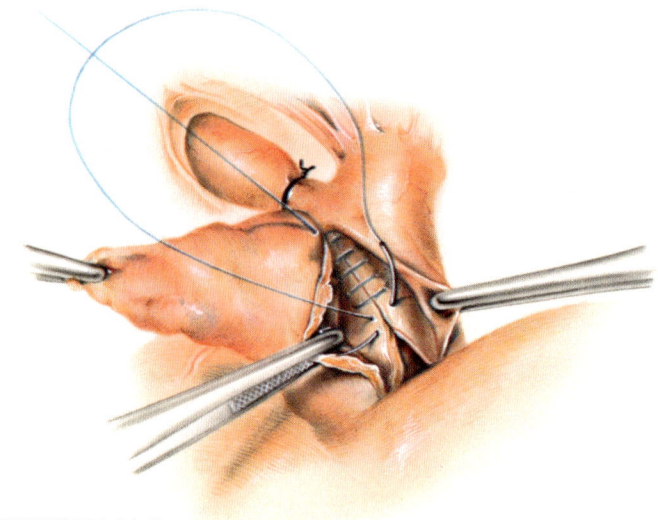

FIGURE 24-5

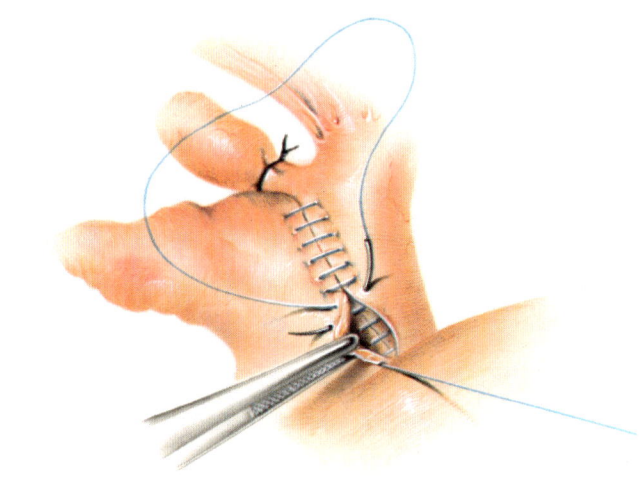

FIGURE 24-6

The posterior suture line is performed from inside, using running suture of 6-0 or 7-0 polypropylene (Fig. 24-5). The anterior row is then performed (Fig. 24-6). The atrial septal defect is closed through the right atrium.

Cardiac Type

Surgical Anatomy
The pulmonary veins empty into a greatly enlarged coronary sinus (Fig. 24-7). A foramen ovale defect is present. Mixed types usually have a cardiac component.[8]

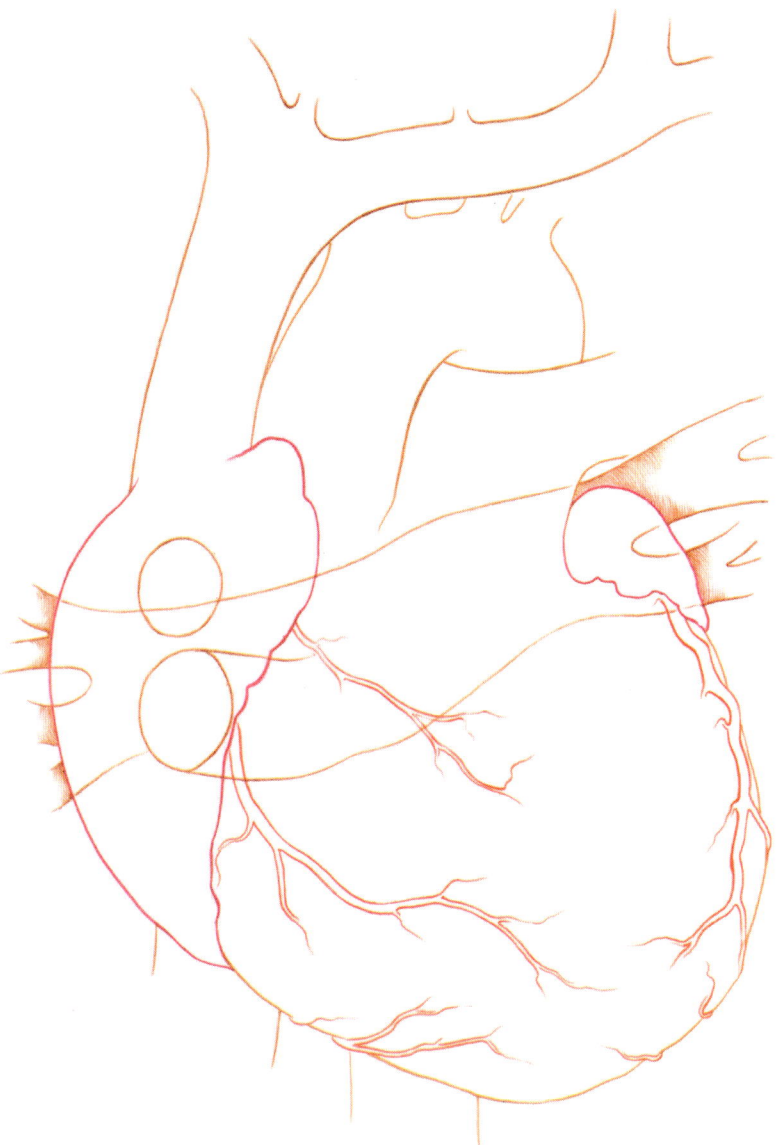

FIGURE 24-7

Surgical Technique

The technique is a modification of that described by Van Praagh and colleagues.[30] The wall between the coronary sinus and the left atrium is everted with a right-angle clamp (Fig. 24-8) and excised through the foramen ovale. The foramen ovale is then closed primarily and the coronary sinus is covered with a Dacron patch (Fig. 24-9).

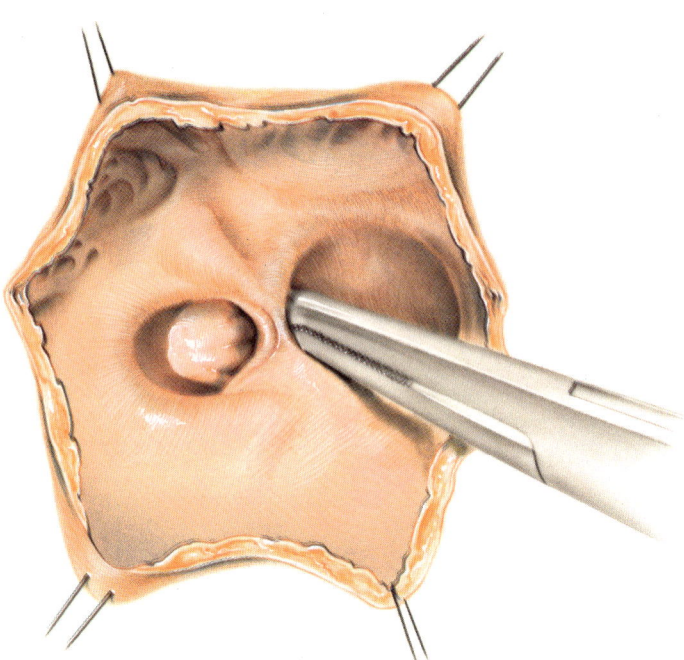

FIGURE 24-8

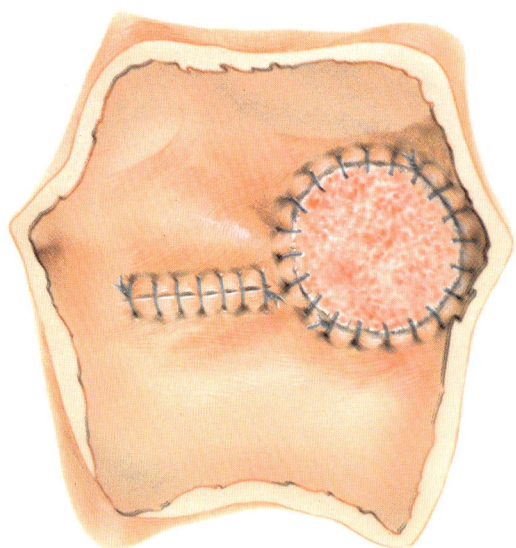

FIGURE 24-9

Infracardiac Type

Surgical Anatomy
Infracardiac TAPVC connects below the diaphragm (Fig. 24-10). Approximately 70% connect to the portal vein; other connections are to the inferior vena cava, ductus venosus, or hepatic vein.[10] In rare instances the only connection may be via collaterals in the azygos system.[18] In some instances the common pulmonary venous trunk can be quite small,[17] and when associated with hypoplasia of the pulmonary veins is uncorrectable.

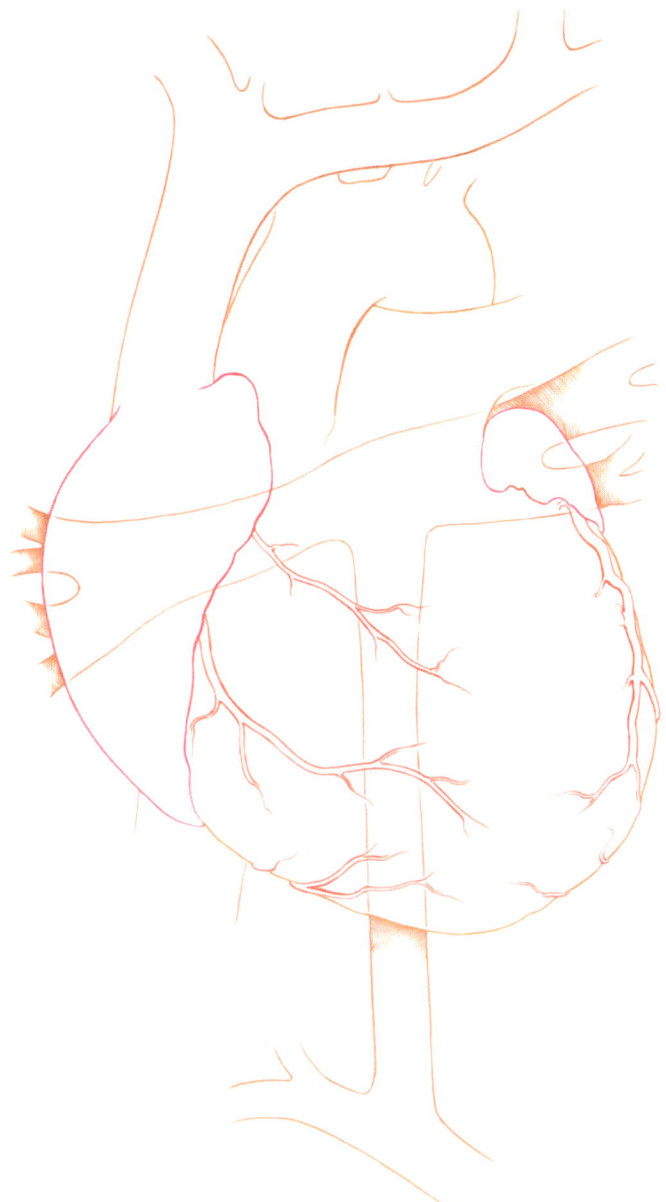

FIGURE 24-10

Surgical Technique
The repair is similar to that for the supracardiac type. The incision in the common pulmonary venous trunk is usually more vertical than horizontal, and may be extended into the vertical vein. The vertical vein is mobilized through the diaphragm to obtain adequate length. It is divided if necessary to avoid tension on the anastomosis. The atrial defect is closed.

Results

Operative mortalities reported in the 1960s and early 1970s were frequently high, from 50% to 65% for patients less than one year[6,33] and as high as 89% for patients less than six months of age.[23] Recent reports have shown dramatic improvement in operative mortality, as low as 13%.[16,29,31] Infracardiac type is associated with a higher operative mortality.[9,10,15,29] The mixed type is often associated with a high mortality in the neonatal period.

Late survival and functional result in patients repaired in childhood are excellent.[5,14] Postoperative hemodynamics are frequently normal following repair in infancy.[20]

Late death following repair in infancy is unusual,[13] but when it occurs a common cause is intimal fibroplasia of the pulmonary veins away from the anastomosis, a syndrome occurring more commonly in the cardiac and infracardiac types.[11,29,31]

References

1. Bharati S, Lev M: Congenital anomalies of the pulmonary veins. Cardiovasc Clin 5:23, 1973.
2. Bonham Carter RE, Capriles M, Noe Y: Total anomalous pulmonary venous drainage: a clinical and anatomical study of 75 children. Br Heart J 31:45, 1969.
3. Bove KE, Geiser EA, Meyer RA: The left ventricle in anomalous pulmonary venous return. Arch Pathol Lab Med 99:522, 1975.
4. Burroughs JT, Edwards JE: Total anomalous pulmonary venous connection. Am Heart J 59:913, 1960.
5. Clarke DR, Stark J, DeLeval M, Pincott JR, Taylor JFN: Total anomalous pulmonary venous drainage in infancy. Br Heart J 39:436, 1977.
6. Cooley DA, Hallman GL: Surgical Treatment of Congenital Heart Disease. Philadelphia, Lea & Febiger, 1966, p 143.
7. Cooley DA, Ochsner A Jr: Correction of total anomalous pulmonary venous drainage: technical considerations. Surgery 42:1014, 1957.
8. DeLeval M, Stark J, Waterston DJ: Mixed type of total anomalous pulmonary venous drainage. Ann Thorac Surg 16:464, 1973.
9. DiEusanio G, Sandrasagra FA, Donnelly RJ, Hamilton DI: Total anomalous pulmonary venous connection. Thorax 33:275, 1978.
10. Duff DF, Nihill MR, McNamara DG: Infradiaphragmatic total anomalous pulmonary venous return: review of clinical and pathological findings and results of operation in 28 cases. Br Heart J 39:619, 1977.
11. Fleming WH, Clark EB, Dooley KJ, Hofschire PJ, Ruckman RN, Hopeman AR, Sarafian L, Mooring PK: Late complications following surgical repair of total anomalous pulmonary venous return below the diaphragm. Ann Thorac Surg 27:435, 1979.
12. Gathman GE, Nadas AS: Total anomalous pulmonary venous connection: clinical and physiologic observations of 75 pediatric patients. Circulation 42:143, 1970.
13. Gersony WM, Bowman FO, Steeg CN, Hayes CJ, Jesse MJ, Malm JR: Management of total anomalous pulmonary venous drainage in early infancy. Circulation 43(Suppl I):I-19, 1971.
14. Gomes MMR, Feldt RH, McGoon DC, Danielson GK: Long-term results following correction of total anomalous pulmonary venous connection. J Thorac Cardiovasc Surg 61:253, 1971.
15. Higashino SM, Shaw GG, May IA, Ecker RR: Total anomalous pulmonary venous drainage below the diaphragm: clinical presentation, hemodynamic findings, and surgical results. J Thorac Cardiovasc Surg 68:711, 1974.
16. Katz NM, Kirklin JW, Pacifico AD: Concepts and practices in surgery for total anomalous pulmonary venous connection. Ann Thorac Surg 25:479, 1978.

17. Kawashima Y, Matsuda H, Nakano S, Miyamoto K, Fujino M, Kozuka T, Manabe H: Tree-shaped pulmonary veins in infracardiac total anomalous pulmonary venous drainage. Ann Thorac Surg 23:436, 1977.
18. Khonsari S, Starr A: Unpublished data.
19. Kirklin JW: Surgical treatment of total anomalous pulmonary venous connection in infancy. *In* Barratt-Boyes BG, Neutze JM, Harris EA (eds): Heart Disease in Infancy, Diagnosis and Surgical Treatment. Edinburgh and London, Churchill/Livingstone, 1973, p 89.
20. Mathew R, Thilenius OG, Replogle RL, Arcilla RA: Cardiac function in total anomalous pulmonary venous return before and after surgery. Circulation 55:361, 1977.
21. Muller WH: The surgical treatment of transposition of the pulmonary veins. Ann Surg 134:683, 1951.
22. Mullins CE, El-Said G, Neches WH, Williams RL, Vargo TA, Nihill MR, McNamara DG: Balloon atrial septostomy for total anomalous pulmonary venous return. Br Heart J 35:752, 1973.
23. Mustard WT, Keon WJ, Trusler GA: Transposition of the lesser veins (total anomalous pulmonary venous drainage). Prog Cardiovasc Dis 11:145, 1968.
24. Parr GVS, Kirklin JW, Pacifico AD, Blackstone EH, Lauridsen P: Cardiac performance in infants after repair of total anomalous pulmonary venous connection. Ann Thorac Surg 17:561, 1974.
25. Roe BB: Posterior approach to correction of total anomalous pulmonary venous return: further experience. J Thorac Cardiovasc Surg 59:748, 1970.
26. Roe BB: Total anomalous pulmonary venous drainage, technical and physiological considerations. Ann Surg 160:1, 1964.
27. Shumacker HB Jr, King H: A modified procedure for complete repair of total anomalous pulmonary venous drainage. Surg Gynecol Obstet 112:763, 1961.
28. Tucker BL, Lindesmith GG, Stiles QR, Meyer BW: The superior approach for correction of the supracardiac type of total anomalous pulmonary venous return. Ann Thorac Surg 22:374, 1976.
29. Turley K, Tucker WY, Ullyot DJ, Ebert PA: Total anomalous pulmonary venous connection in infancy: influence of age and type of lesion. Am J Cardiol 45:92, 1980.
30. Van Praagh R, Harken AH, Delisle G, Ando M, Gross RE: Total anomalous pulmonary venous drainage to the coronary sinus. J Thorac Cardiovasc Surg 64:132, 1972.
31. Whight CM, Barratt-Boyes BG, Calder AL, Neutze JM, Brandt PWT: Total anomalous pulmonary venous connection: long-term results following repair in infancy. J Thorac Cardiovasc Surg 75:52, 1978.
32. Williams GR, Richardson WR, Campbell GS: Repair of total anomalous pulmonary venous drainage in infancy. J Thorac Cardiovasc Surg 47:199, 1964.
33. Wukasch DC, Deutsch M, Reul GJ, Hallman GL, Cooley DA: Total anomalous pulmonary venous return: review of 125 patients treated surgically. Ann Thorac Surg 19:622, 1975.

Index

A
Abscess, aortic root, 212–13
Afterload mismatch, 224
Aneurysm, left ventricular, 233–39
  angina pectoris and, 234
  arrhythmias and, 234
  congestive failure and, 233–34
  coronary artery disease and, 235
  diagnosis, 233
  embolism and, systemic, 235
  mitral regurgitation and, 235
  plication, 233
  resection, 233–39
    anatomy and, 235
    indications, 233–35
    mortality, 234, 238
    results, 238–39
    strategy, 235
    survival, 239
    technique, 235–38
  "true" vs. "false," 233
Angina pectoris
  aneurysm and, left ventricular, 234
  aortic stenosis and, 207
Anticoagulation
  aortic valve replacement and, 210, 225
  morbidity and mortality, 225
Anuloplasty, tricuspid valve, 247–52
  anatomy and, 248–49
  choice of technique, 248
  indications, 247–48
  results, 252
  strategy, 248
  techniques, 249–51
    Carpentier ring, 250–51
    DeVega, 249–50
Anulus, aortic, 211–13, 219, 223

Aorta
  balloon pump in, septal rupture and, 242–43
  pulmonary artery ratio to, 289
  transposition of. See Transposition of great arteries.
  Waterston shunt and, 290
Aortic valve, 205–26
  anatomy, 205, 213–14
  area index, 208
  calcification, 216–18
  commissures, 205
  endocarditis and, 209–10, 212
  gradient, 208
  incisions, 205, 206, 215–16
  insufficiency, ventricular septal defect and, 277–78
  membrane, subaortic, 226
  regurgitation, 208–9, 224
    stenosis combined with, 209
  replacement, 206–26
    abscesses and, 212–13
    anatomy and, 213–14
    complications, prosthesis-related, 225
    coronary artery surgery and, 210, 211
    enlargement of anulus and, 223
    erosion and, anular, 212–13
    indications, 206–10
    mitral valve replacement and, 211
    mortality, 224
    myocardial preservation and, 211
    prostheses for, 210–11, 225
    results, 224–25
    small anulus and, 211–12
    strategy, 211–13
    survival after, late, 224

    suturing in, 211, 218–22
    technique, 215–23
    thromboembolism after, 225
    venting and, 211
    ventricular function after, 224
  sizing of anulus of, 219
  stenosis, 205, 206–8, 224
    idiopathic hypertrophic subaortic (IHSS), 226
    membranous subvalvular, 226
    regurgitation and, 209
    supravalvular, 226
    tetralogy of Fallot and, 297
Aortic valvotomy, 205–6
  anatomy and, 205
  indications, 205
  results, 206
  technique, 206
Aortic valvuloplasty, 278
Aortotomy
  closure of, 223
  transverse, 206, 215
Aortoventriculoplasty, 212
Arrhythmias
  aortic stenosis and, 207
  atrial, Mustard operation and, 305, 314
  endocardial excision for, 239
  Senning operation and, 321
  tetralogy of Fallot repair and, 299
  ventricular, aneurysms and, 234, 239
Atrial septal defects, 261–67
  AV canal defect and, 270
  indications for surgery, 261
  ostium primum, 261, 266–67
  ostium secundum, 261, 264–65
  sinus venosus, 262–63
  TAPVC and, 334, 336
  tetralogy of Fallot and, 291

343

Index

Atrial septectomy, 304
Atrial septostomy, 304
Atriotomy
  Mustard operation and, 309
  right, 262
  Senning operation and, 317, 318
  ventricular septal defect repair and, 281
Atrioventricular bundle. *See* Bundle of His.
Atrioventricular canal, complete, 269–74
  AV valves and, 270
  conduction system and, 270
  indications for surgery, 269
  results of repair of, 274
  septal defect in, 270
  surgical anatomy, 270
  surgical strategy, 269
  surgical technique, 270–74
  tetralogy of Fallot and, 291
  ventricular size and dominance and, 270
Atrioventricular node, 249
  AV canal defect and, 270, 272
  Mustard operation and, 314
  ventricular septal defect and, 279
Atrioventricular valves. *See also* Mitral valve; Tricuspid valve.
  anterior common leaflet and, 270
Atrium
  left
    Mustard operation and, 307, 309
    Senning operation and, 318
    TAPVC and, 334, 335, 338
  right
    Mustard operation and, 307, 313
    Senning operation and, 317–18, 321
    TAPVC and, 334, 336
Azygos vein
  sinus venosus defect and, 262
  TAPVC and, 339

B

Baffle, Mustard operation, 307–11, 316
Balloon atrial septostomy, 304
Balloon pump, intraaortic, septal rupture repair and, 242–43
Ball-valve prostheses, 210
  comparison of, 225
  fit of, 219
  thromboembolism and, 225
  tricuspid valve, 252
Banding, pulmonary artery, 269
  transposition and, 323
  ventricular septal defect and, 277, 285
Bioprosthesis. *See also* Porcine valve.
Bjork-Shiley valve, 225
Blalock-Hanlon septectomy, 304
Blalock-Taussig shunt, 290
  transposition of great arteries and, 323
Block, heart
  Mustard operation and, 314
  tetralogy of Fallot repair and, 299

Bundle branch block, right, tetralogy of Fallot and, 299
Bundle of His, 249
  AV canal defect and, 270
  tetralogy of Fallot and, 292–93
  ventricular septal defect and, 279

C

Calcification, aortic valve, 216–18
Cardiopulmonary bypass
  aneurysmectomy and, ventricular, 235
  transposition of great arteries and, 306
  ventricular septal defect repair and, 277
Carpentier ring anuloplasty, 250–51
Central fibrous body, 249
  tetralogy of Fallot and, 293
  ventricular septal defect and, 279
Cerebrovascular accident, transposition of great arteries and, 304
Chordae tendineae
  aneurysmectomy and, ventricular, 237
  AV canal defects and, 270, 272
  tricuspid valve and, 248, 253
  ventricular septal defect and, 283
Commissures
  aortic valve, 205
  pulmonary valve, 259, 294
  tricuspid valve, 249–52
Commissurotomy
  pulmonary, 294
  tricuspid valve, 252
Conduction system
  AV canal defects and, 270
  tetralogy of Fallot and, 292
  ventricular septal defect and, 279–80
Conoventricular septal defect, 279
Contractility, aortic valve replacement and, 224
Conus septum, tetralogy of Fallot and, 294
Coronary arteries
  anterior descending, 324
    anomaly of, 289, 291
  circumflex, 324, 327
  right, 324
    aortotomy and, 215
  transposition of great arteries and, 305, 321, 324, 325, 327
  ventricular septal defect repair and, 243, 284
Coronary artery bypass
  aneurysmectomy and, ventricular, 235
  aortic valve replacement and, 210, 211
Coronary sinus
  conduction tissue and, 279–80
  Mustard operation and, 307, 309, 311
  ostium primum defect and, 266
  TAPVC and, 337, 338
Crista supraventricularis
  tetralogy of Fallot and, 294, 297
  ventricular septal defect and, 279, 281

D

Dacron patch
  aortic valve replacement and, 223
  AV canal defect repair and, 272
  Mustard operation and, 307
  ostium secundum repair and, 265
  sinus venosus defect repair and, 262
  TAPVC repair and, 338
  ventricular septal defect repair and, 243–45, 281, 282, 284, 295
Debridement, aortic valve calcification and, 217, 218
DeVega anuloplasty, 249–50
Dilators, pulmonary stenosis and, 291
Double-patch technique, ventricular septal defect repair by, 243
Ductus arteriosus, patent, transposition of great arteries and, 307
Ductus venosus, TAPVC and, 339
Dysrhythmia. *See* Arrhythmias.

E

Echocardiography, aortic regurgitation and, 209
Ejection fraction
  aneurysmectomy and, 234, 239
  aortic regurgitation and, 208, 209, 224
  aortic stenosis and, 224
Electrophysiology
  Mustard operation and, 314–15
  Senning operation and, 321
  tetralogy of Fallot repair and, 299
Embolism, aortic valve prostheses and, 225
Endocardial cushions, ostium primum defect and, 266
Endocardial excision, 239
Endocarditis, aortic valve replacement and, 209–10, 212
Erosions, aortic root, 212–13
Eustachian valve, Senning operation and, 317, 321

F

Fallot's tetralogy. *See* Tetralogy of Fallot.
Fibroplasia, intimal, of pulmonary veins, 340
Fibrous body, central, 249, 279, 293
Foramen ovale
  pulmonary stenosis and, 257
  TAPVC and, 334, 337, 338
Fossa ovalis, 262

H

Hancock xenograft, 225
Heart failure, congestive
  aneurysm and, left ventricular, 233–34
  aortic valve replacement and, 206, 207
  aortic valvotomy and, 205
  AV canal defects and, 269
  ventricular septal defects and, 276

Hemiblock, left anterior, tetralogy of
    Fallot repair and, 299
Hepatic vein, TAPVC and, 339
His bundle. *See* Bundle of His.
Hypertension, pulmonary
    atrial septal defect and, 261
    ventricular septal defect and, 276
Hypertrophic subaortic stenosis,
    idiopathic (IHSS), 226
Hypertrophy, left ventricular
    aortic regurgitation and, 208
    aortic stenosis and, 206, 207, 224
Hypoxemia
    tetralogy of Fallot and, 289
    transposition of great arteries and, 304

I
Iben's double-patch technique, 243
IHSS (idiopathic hypertrophic subaortic
    stenosis), 226
Incisions
    aneurysmectomy, ventricular, 237
    aortic valve, 205, 206, 215–16
    AV canal defect repair, 270–71
    Mustard operation, 309, 313
    Senning operation, 317, 318
    TAPVC repair, 335
    tetralogy of Fallot repair, 293–95
    tricuspid commissurotomy, 252
    ventricular septal defect repair, 280–85
Infundibular stenosis
    pulmonary valvotomy and, 257–58
    tetralogy of Fallot and, 289, 293, 298
Innominate vein, TAPVC and, 334
Instruments, pulmonary valvotomy, 258–59
Intimal fibroplasia, pulmonary vein, 339
Intraaortic balloon pump, septal rupture
    repair and, 242–43

K
Koch's triangle, 279–80

L
Laplace relationship, 234

M
Membranous septum, ventricular septal
    defect and, 279, 282
Membranous subvalvular aortic stenosis,
    226
Mitral valve
    AV canal defect and, 272
    Mustard operation and, 309
    ostium primum defect and, 266
    replacement
        aneurysmectomy and, ventricular, 235
        aortic valve replacement and, 211

Mustard operation, 303, 305, 307–16
    electrophysiology after, 314–15
    hemodynamics after, 315–16
    palliative, 306
    reoperation after, 307
    results, 314–16
    technique, 307–13
Myectomy, transaortic, 226
Myocardial infarction
    aneurysm and, left ventricular, 233, 234, 235
    ventricular septal defect and, 242–45
Myocardial ischemia
    aneurysm and, left ventricular, 234
    aortic stenosis and, 207
Myocardium
    akinetic, 233
    degeneration of aortic regurgitation
        and, 208–9
    preservation of
        aneurysmectomy and, 235
        aortic valve replacement and, 211
        pulmonary valvotomy and, 257
        tricuspid anuloplasty and, 248
    sinusoids in, 256
Myofibrils, aortic regurgitation and, 208–9

O
Ostium primum defects, 261, 266–67
    anatomy, 266
    AV canal defect and, 270
    results of repair, 266
    technique of repair, 266, 267
Ostium secundum defects, 261
    results of repair, 265
    surgical anatomy, 264
    surgical technique, 264–65

P
Papillary muscles
    aneurysmectomy and, ventricular, 237
    AV canal defects and, 270
    tricuspid valve and, 248
    ventricular septal defect and, 283
Pars membranacea, ventricular septal
    defect and, 292
Patch. *See also* Dacron patch.
    transanular, 257, 290–91, 298
Patent ductus arteriosus, transposition of
    great arteries and, 307
Plication
    aneurysmal, 233
    tricuspid anulus, 250, 251
Porcine valves, 210, 225
    durability of, 225
    thromboembolism and, 225
Portal vein, TAPVC and, 339
Potts anastomosis, 290
Premature ventricular contractions,
    tetralogy of Fallot repair and, 299

Propranolol, tetralogy of Fallot and, 288–89
Prostaglandin E_1, pulmonary stenosis
    and, 256
Prostheses
    aortic valve, 210–11, 225
    ball-valve, 210, 219, 225, 252
    Bjork-Shiley, 225
    comparisons of, 225
    complications of, 225
    Hancock xenograft, 225
    hemodynamics, 225
    porcine, 210, 225
    Starr-Edwards, 210, 219, 225
    structural failure of, 225
    thromboembolism and, 225
    tilting-disc, 225, 252
    tricuspid valve, 252
Pseudoaneurysm, ventricular, 233
Pulmonary artery
    banding
        AV canal defects and, 269
        transposition and, 323
        ventricular septal defect and, 277, 285
    hypoplasia, tetralogy of Fallot and, 289
    single, 291
    transposition. *See* Transposition of
        great arteries.
Pulmonary hypertension
    atrial septal defect and, 261
    ventricular septal defect and, 276
Pulmonary-systemic shunts, 290
Pulmonary valve
    absent, 291
    commissurotomy, 294
    minimum ring diameter, 291
    stenosis, 256–59
        assessment of, 291
        tetralogy of Fallot and, 289, 293, 294
        transposition of great arteries and, 306, 323, 325
    transanular patch, 257, 290–91, 298
    ventricular septal defect and, 279
Pulmonary valvotomy, 256–59
    in child or adult, 257, 259
    closed, 258–59
    foramen ovale and, 257
    indications, 256–57
    infundibular resection in, 257–58
    instruments for, 258–59
    in neonate, 256–57, 259
    open, 259
    results, 259
    strategy, 257–58
    technique, 258–59
    transanular patch in, 257
Pulmonary vascular disease
    AV canal defects and, 269
    transposition of great arteries and, 304, 306
    ventricular septal defects and, 276
Pulmonary veins
    intimal fibroplasia of, 339

Pulmonary veins *(cont'd)*
  Mustard operation and, 309–11, 313, 316
  Senning operation and, 318, 321
  sinus venosus defect and, 262
  total anomalous connection of (TAPVC), 333–40
    anatomy, 334, 337, 339
    cardiac type of, 337–38
    indications for surgery, 333
    infracardiac type of, 339
    results of repair of, 340
    strategy for, surgical, 333
    supracardiac type of, 333–36
    technique of repair of, 334–36, 338–39
Pump function
  aortic regurgitation and, 209, 224
  aortic stenosis and, 206–7

R
Rashkind septostomy, 304
Rastelli classification of AV valves, 270
Rastelli operation, 306
Ring anuloplasty, Carpentier, 250–51
Rongeurs, aortic valve calcification and, 217

S
Saline, cold, AV canal defect repair and, 270
Secundum defects. *See* Ostium secundum defects.
Senning operation, 303, 305, 317–21
  results, 321
  technique, 317–21
Septectomy, atrial, 304
Septostomy, balloon atrial, 304
Shunts
  Blalock-Taussig, 290, 323
  left-to-right
    atrial septal defect and, 261
    AV canal defects and, 269
    ventricular septal defect and, 276
  right-to-left
    pulmonary stenosis and, 257
    tetralogy of Fallot and, 292
  systemic-pulmonary, 290
  tetralogy of Fallot and, 290
  Waterston, 290
Sinus node
  Mustard operation and, 314–15
  sinus venosus defect and, 262, 263
Sinus venosus defect, 262–63
  anatomy, 262
  results, 263
  surgical technique, 262–63
Sizers
  aortic valve, 219
  tricuspid valve, 250
Staphylococcal endocarditis, 209–10, 212

Starr-Edwards valve, 210
  comparison of, 225
  fit of, 219
  thromboembolism and, 225
Sternotomy, median, TAPVC repair and, 334
Stress, aortic regurgitation and, 209
Subclavian artery, systemic-pulmonary shunts and, 290
Suture technique
  aneurysmectomy, ventricular, 237–38
  aortic valve replacement, 211, 218–22
  AV canal defect repair and, 272–74
  Carpentier ring anuloplasty, 251
  DeVega anuloplasty, 249
  Mustard operation, 307–13
  ostium primum defect repair, 266
  ostium secundum closure, 265
  Senning operation, 318–21
  sinus venosus defect repair, 262, 263
  TAPVC repair, 336
  tetralogy of Fallot repair, 295–97
  ventricular septal defect repair, 244, 281–84
Systemic-pulmonary shunts, 290

T
Tachycardia, ventricular, endocardial excision for, 239
TAPVC. *See* Pulmonary veins, total anomalous connection of.
Tendon of Todaro, 279–80
Tetralogy of Fallot, 288–99
  anatomy, 292–93
  anomalies associated with, 291
  conduction system and, 292–93
  electrophysiology, 299
  hemodynamic status and, 289, 299
  indications for surgery, 288–89
  infundibular stenosis and, 289, 293, 298
  palliation, 290
    initial, vs. primary total correction, 288–89
  propranolol for, 288–89
  pulmonic stenosis and, 289, 293, 294
  reoperation, 289
  results of repair of, 298–99
  shunt closure, 290
  strategy for, surgical, 290–92
  technique of repair, 293–98
  transanular patch and, 290–91, 298
  ventricular septal defect and, 292, 295
Thromboembolism, prostheses and, aortic valve, 225
Thrombus
  mural, ventricular aneurysm and, 235
  tricuspid prosthesis and, 252
Tilting-disc valve
  comparison of, 225
  thromboembolism and, 225
  tricuspid, 252
Todaro's tendon, 279–80

Total anomalous pulmonary venous connection. *See* Pulmonary veins, total anomalous connection of.
Transanular patch
  pulmonary stenosis and, 257
  tetralogy of Fallot and, 290–91, 298
Transposition of great arteries, 303–28
  anatomic correction of, 303, 305, 321–28
    anatomy, 324
    preparation of left ventricle, 323
    results, 328
    technique, 325–27
  atrial septectomy for, 304
  balloon atrial septostomy for, 304
  cerebrovascular accident and, 304
  choice of operation, 305–6
  historical note on, 303
  indications for surgery, 303–5
  inflow vs. outflow procedure for, 305
  Mustard operation for, 303, 305, 307–16
    electrophysiology after, 314–15
    hemodynamics after, 315–16
    results, 314–16
    technique, 307–13
  patent ductus arteriosus and, 307
  pulmonary stenosis and, 306
  pulmonary vascular disease and, 304
  Rastelli operation for, 306
  reoperation for, 307
  Senning operation for, 303, 305, 317–21
    results, 321
    technique, 317–21
  strategy for, surgical, 306–7
  ventricular septal defect and, 306
Triangle of Koch, 279–80
Tricuspid valve, 247–53
  anuloplasty, 247–52
    anatomy and, 248–49
    Carpentier ring, 250–51
    choice of technique, 248
    DeVega, 249–50
    indications, 247–48
    results, 252
    strategy, 248
    techniques, 249–51
  commissurotomy, 252
    indications and technique, 252
  insufficiency, 247, 250, 252, 253
  regurgitation, 247–48
  replacement, 247, 253
    indications and strategy, 253
    technique and results, 253
  stenosis, 252
  tetralogy of Fallot and, 297
  transposition of great arteries and, 305, 309, 311, 315, 316
  ventricular septal defect and, 284
Trigone, right fibrous, 249

V

Valves, prosthetic. *See* Prostheses.
Valvotomy
  aortic, 205–6
  pulmonary, 256–59
Valvuloplasty, aortic, 278
Vena cava
  inferior
    Mustard operation and, 311, 316
    ostium secundum defect and, 264, 265
    Senning operation and, 318, 321
    TAPVC and, 339
  superior
    Mustard operation and, 311, 316
    Senning operation and, 318, 321
    sinus venosus defect and, 262
    systemic-pulmonary shunts and, 290
Venting
  aneurysmectomy and, ventricular, 237, 238
  aortic valve replacement and, 211
Ventricle
  AV canal defects and, 270
  failure. *See* Heart failure.
  left
    aneurysm of. *See* Aneurysm, left ventricular.
    compensation, 206–7, 208
    dilatation, 208
    filling pressure, 239
    hypertrophy, 206, 207, 208, 224
    pressure, 206
    rupture, 233
    TAPVC and, 334
    transposition of great arteries and, 305, 306, 323
  right
    classification of, 278–79
    pressure, 257
    pulmonary stenosis and, 256
    transposition of great arteries and, 305, 316
    types of, 256
Ventricular septal defects, 276–85
  anatomy, 278–80
  aortic insufficiency and, 277–78
  AV canal defect and, 270
  choice of operation, 277
  conduction system and, 279–80
  indications for surgery, 276–77
  location of defect, 278–79
  membranous type, 279, 282
  muscular, 279, 284
  posterior, 279, 283–84
  postinfarction, repair of, 242–45
    anatomy and, 243
    anteroapical defect closure, 243–44
    balloon pump and, intraaortic, 242–43
    coronary artery disease and, 243
    indications, 242
    mitral regurgitation and, 243
    results, 245
    strategy, 242–43
    technique, 243–45
  pulmonary artery banding and, 277, 285
  results of repair of, 285
  supracristal type, 279, 281
  surgical strategy, 277–78
  technique of repair, 280–85
  tetralogy of Fallot and, 292, 295
  transposition of great arteries and, 306
Ventricular tachycardia, endocardial excision for, 239
Ventriculotomy
  septal defect repair and, 243, 245, 280–81, 284
  tetralogy of Fallot and, 293–95
Vertical vein, left, TAPVC and, 334, 335, 339

W

Waterston shunt, 290

X

Xenografts, procine. *See* Porcine valves.

Ricardo Navas